Taking care of my wife Rakhi with Parkinson's

Dilip Guha

This book is dedicated to the memory of my beloved wife, Dr. Chandralekha (Rakhi) Guha, whom I loved dearly and unconditionally, and provided my all humanly possible support during her illness of almost 10 years until her passing after a long battle of Parkinson's disease. I feel deeply that I was placed in this world to serve my wife. She was my soul mate. I will miss her forever.

Acknowledgements

Though I kept a diary of my experience during last ten (10) years of my wife's illness before she expired after a long battle of Parkinson's disease, I was not sure whether I wanted to publish my memoir. Later, I realized that it would be a good idea to share my experience with the patients, the families, and the caregivers in the similar situation so that they could be benefited from this biography.

A friend in need is a friend indeed. Through this difficult time I came to know who my real friends were. I came across many acquaintances and friends during my past 40 years through my social and professional activities. But I was able to count on few of them who would not pass judgments unnecessarily and come forward to help or support especially when I was going through difficult times. I would be remiss to write this book and not mention their names. Some of these friends are Panna Dhar, Pronoy Chatterjee and Anarkali Sarkar, Chitralekha Pal, Binita Dutta, Pushpita Bandopadhya, Arati Bhattacharya and their family members.

I like to thank Dr. Pronoy Chatterjee who encouraged me to write this memoir. I also like to thank Ms. Sushmita Dutt who helped me to translate some of Rakhi's poems from Bengali to English.

I am proud of my daughter, Koel, and my son, Roni, for what they had to go through and how they handled the difficult situations as family members, which still affect us in our daily lives. I am also lucky to receive unconditional love and unwavering support from my daughter (Koel), my son-in-law (Sanjeev) and my son (Roni).

My Childhood

At the age of almost sixty, when I look back at my life, I'm fascinated by the challenges and experiences I have gone through. My father was a medical doctor from Calcutta University and worked as civil surgeon for the government of East Pakistan (now Bangladesh). In 1950, as Bengal was partitioned by the British into East and West Bengal, my mother left East Bengal and migrated to Calcutta with her eight children, leaving my father behind. Though my father used to earn reasonably good money, we lived a middle-class life because my mother had to raise a large family (I was the youngest).

My mother was a very hardworking lady who made sure we had the right education from the beginning. By the time we were in middle and high school, my mother, like other parents, closely watched us and continuously pushed and encouraged so we were always at the top of the class and could become doctors. I graduated first in my class from high school. I was awarded a national merit scholarship for which I did not have to pay any expenses for my education. In addition, I got 120 Rupees per month from the government while I attended the engineering college. Though it was a not lot of money, my mother was happy when I handed this money over to her.

Though my parents wanted me to follow in my father's footsteps and become a doctor, I had a natural knack for mathematics and attended engineering college (Jadavpur University) to become an electrical engineer. I was one of the top students and graduated successfully with first class honors and a gold medal. After working a few years in India, I immigrated to the USA for higher education, and the rest is history.

Rakhi's Childhood

My wife, Chandralekha (nicknamed Rakhi), was born in Calcutta in a middle-class, educated family. She was good-looking and the youngest of three children. Her brother was a handsome and intelligent man who graduated from Indian Institute of Technology (IIT), Kharagpur. He loved Rakhi very much and gave her nick name after Raksha Bandhan (Rakhi) festival, which is the celebration of the perfect bond of care between a brother and a sister in Hindu religion. When Rakhi heard the news that her brother had died suddenly of a heart attack at the early age of sixty, she was ill and did not say much except she uttered that she had lost the man who loved her the most and she was closest to in her life. Her sister, Chitralekha (Khuku) came to the USA long before Rakhi arrived, and she has lived in Los Angeles for the last forty years.

Rakhi did not show much interest in studies at an early age but improved significantly in high school. At her mother's insistence, she went to medical school to follow her father's footsteps. He was a medical doctor and a professor at R. G. Kar Medical College, Calcutta, India.

Rakhi graduated in 1980 as a medical doctor with a specialization in pediatrics from Calcutta National Medical College. As a foreign medical graduate, Rakhi had to overcome many hurdles, but she was determined to pursue her career in medicine. She worked hard and finally completed her residency in neurology and psychiatry from New York University in 1991. She went on to complete an EEG fellowship from UMDNJ and joined a practice in Edison, New Jersey, in 1992. Three years later, Rakhi started a solo practice and worked diligently to establish herself as a committed and successful neurologist in the community.

Travel to New York

I was very excited to hear the announcement from the pilot that our plane was finally landing at JFK airport on the evening of August 15, 1975, which originally started at Bombay (now Mumbai), about twenty-four hours ago. I was looking through the window at the ground and was amazed to watch as the whole of New York City glittered by the shower of bright lights. This was my first time traveling by air to a foreign country, and I had never experienced a spectacular sight like this before.

I graduated from Jadavpur University at Kolkata (formerly Calcutta) in electrical engineering in 1971. Immediately after my graduation, I was hired by Calcutta Electric Supply as a GOI trainee. After working there for about six months, I got my first job at Defense Research Development Laboratory (DRDL) at Hyderabad, Andhra Pradesh. But after staying there for two weeks, I went to Bombay to work for Bhaba Atomic Research Center. I could not survive there long, as I felt homesick being on my own for the first time in my life. As a result, I came back to Calcutta to join Garden Reach Workshops after one year. After I came to Calcutta, I made up my mind to go to the USA for higher education. After four years of persistent efforts, I got a call for an interview from the US consulate office and obtained a visa to come to the USA.

I was picked up by my friends, Partha and Sudhir, whom I know from my engineering college, at the airport and taken to Clinton Arms Hotel in Manhattan. I shared an apartment with another immigrant from my state. Half of the money I carried with me went toward the weekly rental fee of sixty dollars. Staying at this hotel had some advantages and disadvantages. Though the hotel was right on Broadway at Ninety-Sixth Street, it was not safe to stay outside at night, and I had to watch over my shoulder while going into and coming out of the hotel. The new immigrants stayed at this hotel because they could not afford expensive places and could mingle with the people of their own background and avoid the impact of the sudden cultural shock. However, it was noisy and filthy, and we literally had to live with cockroaches. Usually, the new immigrants used this hotel as a temporary stop before they became financially solvent and moved to better places.

I was hard-pressed to find a job within a week so that I could survive. I had two choices. I could attend Rensselaer Polytechnic Institute (RPI) in upstate New York, where I had admission with some promise of financial help for the second semester. Or I could find a job with the work permit I had with the immigration visa. But because of my financial situation, I had no choice but to give up my educational goal for the time being and to look for a job in Manhattan. Within a couple of days, I went to an agency to find a job. After an easy test, I landed a job with Chase Manhattan Bank in the check processing department, making minimum wage (five dollars an hour). I was thrilled to know that I would be able to live with two hundred dollars a week, which allowed me to save fifty dollars after paying for my rent and food. I used to stop by McDonald's at the subway station almost every evening for my dinner on the way back to the hotel from work. This was the first time I had eaten beef in my life (by virtue of being born in India, I am Hindu and not supposed to have beef) and started liking the food.

Though I survived for the time being, my goal was to gain higher education. In 1975, the USA was going through a periodic financial downturn, and it was difficult to find a respectable job of reasonable salary with my bachelor's degree in electrical engineering from Jadavpur University. I decided to stay in New York City, and I applied for a master's degree at Columbia University and City College of New York (CCNY). I got the full tuition waived in full at CCNY, and I quit my job at Chase Bank to join CCNY, starting with the spring semester in January 1976. In the summer of 1976, I finished my master's in two semesters with a 4.0 GPA and a thesis. I applied for my PhD at a couple of universities, including Columbia, Berkley, and MIT, while I continued my PhD at CCNY with both student and teaching assistantships.

Though I got admission to MIT, I was interviewed by Bell Labs at the campus and got my dream job at Bell Labs in Whippany, New Jersey, starting on April 4, 1977.

I decided to join Bell Labs as I thought I would end up with an internationally recognized organization like Bell Labs even after I had a degree from MIT. However, I realized later that it was a mistake and a short-sighted decision. I would never forget the day-long interview with several department officers at Bell Labs that continued in the car while riding back to my apartment at Manhattan at the end of the day. I knew that I got the job, and I was so thrilled to realize that my life in the USA had finally started with an annual salary of $19,400.

I was temporarily commuting by bus to go to my work at Whippany from my apartment in Manhattan until I found and moved to my rented apartment in Randolph, New Jersey. I came from the big city of Calcutta, and though NYC was larger than Calcutta, it was not difficult for me to acclimate to Manhattan. At the Clinton Hotel, I was in the midst of so many Indian immigrants that I could imagine I was still in India. Randolph is a remote suburb in northern New Jersey, and I felt suddenly lonely for the first time in the USA.

Before I joined Bell Labs, I started my PhD at CCNY and passed my qualifying examination and began my thesis under Professor Schilling. I was well set in my job. While I was working hard at my job, I continued my PhD program under the Tuition Assistance Plan (TAP), for which I was able to take two days a week off to attend Columbia University for my course work as offered by Bell Labs. I was finally enjoying my independent and bachelor life in America with my friends from my work, engaging in different activities, such as skiing, skating, soccer, and tennis. We even started a soccer club at Whippany.

At my work, I came to know some good friends, like Steve Burtolutii, Mike Burke, Joe Karnacki, and Darlene DuBois, whom I used to invite home for dinner on the weekend. They used to wait for the weekend to have spicy Indian food I cooked for them. Darlene DuBois, whom I dated for a while, finally moved to her home-town, Modesto, California, to take up a teaching job. In the meantime, I visited Calcutta to see my family and to attend my brother's wedding. My parents were offering help to find a girl for me. I decided to find my partner by myself and not to bother and, therefore, involve my old parents.

Marriage

finished my PhD thesis in 1980. After a few years of free and independent bachelor life, I decided to settle down. Though I had arrived at the age of twenty-five, I was slowly but surely becoming part of the American melting pot. However, I realized that I was already molded with Eastern culture and could not be remolded easily with Western culture. Through my friend, I put an advertisement in the *Statesman Newspaper* published in Calcutta and Delhi, looking for a life partner (in those days we did not have social networking websites such as Shadi.com to meet friends). I got several responses and passed them to my parents to have further correspondence.

Finally, I decided to go to India and meet them. My cousin Babli from New Jersey accompanied me to see the family I was mostly interested in. After chatting with family members for almost an hour, I finally met the girl who studied medicine and just finished her internship in pediatrics. After we left, my cousin tried to convince me hard that I must marry the beautiful lady we had just met. I decided not to see anybody else and planned to have dinner with the girl, Chandralekha, alone at the Calcutta

Club to get to know her a little better. We seemed to like each other (love at first sight) and decided to exchange the garland, which is symbol of acceptance of one another in Hindu marriage.

The wedding was set within a few weeks. We were married in a traditional Hindu marriage ceremony (with *sath pake badha*). I remember the first night we were together. She was twenty-eight years old, had never dated a man in her life, and was a little scared to spend the night with a completely unknown man for the first time. I told her not to worry. I had to go back to the USA to work and would need to leave my wife behind until she could get a visa to join me in the near future. I remember I was writing a letter at least once a week, comforting her and assuring her that I was anxious to meet her soon. Within three months, I went to JFK airport to receive my wife with roses. Later she told me that she was not impressed to see me with my tan color and sparkling white teeth. I guess I had been playing soccer and became more tanned than I was before when she saw me for the first time in Calcutta. However, she told me she was impressed with my physical strength when I carried her two heavy suitcases filled with her medical books.

I brought her to Randolph, the remote suburb of New Jersey, where she was lonely without her family and friends. But in a single-bedroom apartment, it did not take a long time for us to get intimate. When I was at work, she spent her time cooking, watching television, and learning to speak with an American accent. Together we used to watch TV shows such as *Family Feud* and enjoyed each other's company and intimacy. I realized she was anxious to start her medical career in the USA as soon as possible.

As a foreign graduate, she would have to pass ECFMG (Educational Commission for Foreign Medical Graduates examination), for which she was ready to take courses at Saint Barnabas Hospital. I still remember the day when she had a very bad experience and became quite upset. I had taken her to Saint Barnabas and was supposed to pick her up after her class at the end of the day. I was waiting for her call. Finally, when I got there to pick her up, she was so upset and scared that she was crying. She wanted to know why I did not to pick her up earlier. I said, "I am sorry. I was waiting for your phone call." She was not satisfied with the answer and never forgot the incident. She complained about the event whenever the matter was brought up in conversation in the future.

She was very unhappy that she would miss the first opportunity to appear for ECFMG in November 1981 and wouldn't make the residency program starting in June 1982. Her best chance was to appear for ECFMG in November 1982 so that she could start her residency in June 1983, a year later. But it did not go according to the plan. She became pregnant, and we had our first baby, a girl, Koel, in September 1982. Rakhi used to get upset when she was asked in the interviews whether she could handle hard work as a resident with a newborn baby. It was then very difficult to get into a residency program. I remember I took her for interviews at almost all the states on the East Coast, such as New Jersey, New York, Connecticut, Rhode Island, Massachusetts, Washington, DC, etc. She had to wait for the residency program in 1983 when our daughter was almost one year old. She was devastated when she found out she was not going to get into the residency program starting in June 1983.

In the meantime, after finishing my PhD, I took a job in the computer department at Bell Labs in Holmdel, New Jersey, and we moved to an apartment in Red Bank, New Jersey. One afternoon I got a frantic call from my wife that our daughter, Koel, was having a seizure. I immediately came home and took her to Riverside Hospital. I had to stay overnight with my daughter to relieve my wife. She was detected of having a benign familial neonatal seizure (BFNS) that happens within several months of birth and do not have serious consequences for a child. We were so relieved to see her out of the danger and back home after several days.

We were enjoying life with our daughter. We moved to our new house in Marlboro, New Jersey, in November 1983.

Residency Training

I t was very difficult at that time for foreign medical graduates to get into a residency program. When my wife found out she was not going to get into the residency program even in June of 1984, she got very upset. I tried to encourage her by involving her in different activities, such as fishing and community services. But it was not good enough. One evening I came home, and I was very scared not to see her there. I was about to call the police. I was so relieved to find her sitting silently behind the door of the Closet. I realized that she was very much depressed.

She decided to visit Calcutta with Koel to see her family for the first time since leaving India. I also thought that it would be a good idea for her to have some type of break. However, she dropped a bombshell when she told me that she was not coming back until and unless she found a job in the USA. I was so concerned that I let her sister in California know and asked her to convince Rakhi otherwise. In the meantime, I was following the correspondence Rakhi had with various hospitals for possible residency opportunities. I was happy to find out that she got an interview for a residency program in Boston. I convinced her to come back, and I was relieved. However, she did not get the job but was interviewed soon at a different hospital and got the residency at Kingsboro Psychiatric Center in Brooklyn, New York, and started her residency in psychiatry in June 1985.

My wife wanted to move to Brooklyn so she could spend more time with our daughter, who was three years old at the time. At the same time, AT&T was going through divestiture, and I was ready to take up an independent consulting job at Bell Labs in Whippany, New Jersey, doubling my salary from fifty thousand dollars to one hundred thousand dollars. I did not want to sell our house in Marlboro, New Jersey, and move to Brooklyn, which would be far from my work.

We finally decided to rent our house in Marlboro and move to Staten Island so that it would be closer to her job. We bought a condo in Staten Island. When we both went to work, we used to drop our daughter off with a Philippine nanny who was very nice. My daughter started going to preschool and eventually to catholic primary school in Staten Island. Finally we were enjoying our married life, watching our sweet and beautiful daughter grow. She was taking lessons for ballet dancing. Though we had long working hours, we made sure that Koel was happy.

After finishing her residency in psychiatry, my wife joined NYU for another three years to complete her second residency in neurology. A joint degree in both neurology and psychiatry would give her more opportunities in her career. We were having problems with the tenants who were not paying rent on our house in Marlboro. We, therefore, decided to sell the condo in Staten Island and move back to our house in 1988. My wife was not thrilled about the move. I could not resist buying a Mercedes car with the money I made by selling the condo. Because of the heavy workload during residency, Rakhi decided to share an apartment in New York with some Philippine nurses while she attended NYU for her second residency. She used to come home on the weekends to spend time with Koel and I.

In the meantime we tried to have more children, but with no success. Rakhi had a couple of miscarriages. In the end, she had no intention of having any more kids, as she was busy with her work. I tried to convince her to have one more child so that Koel would have a sibling to spend time with when she was a grown-up. I was happy when I found out that Rakhi was pregnant. She used to keep herself quite busy and enjoyed gardening and spending time with the family when she was at home on the weekends. Sometimes I was worried, and I used to tell her to take it easy, as she was pregnant.

My mother-in-law came from India to visit us and had helped us take care of our daughter when we were in Staten Island. She came again to help out when my wife was doing her residency at NYU. My daughter became very close to her grandmother when my wife and I were busy and could not spend much time at home because of our workloads. My wife's younger uncle worked as an engineer at Air India and used to fly to New York on a regular basis. He was always accompanied by his wife, Mani, who was very polite. They used to stay with us and also became very close to my daughter.

Business Venture

While I was working at AT&T as a consultant, I eventually became an independent consultant and started a company that supplied consultants to AT&T. I was doing reasonably well financially. Also, on the side, I started working on one of my product ideas at home: PC-based test equipment for telecommunication industries. We designed a high speed T1 interface card that would sit on the ISA bus and diagnose primarily three lower layers (levels one, two, and three) of communication protocol. My friend Rez was mostly involved in the hardware, and I was mostly involved in the software design. I worked extremely hard, frequently going to bed late at night while I was in Staten Island and also when I moved back to New Jersey.

Our Son with Cerebral Palsy

A s my wife was pregnant in her late age, we decided to have an amniocentesis test, which did not show any problem. Rakhi was admitted earlier to the hospital as she was dehydrated, and the doctor advised to have a cesarean. Our second child, Roni (Ranadeb), was born on September 24, 1991. When he was six months old, my wife realized that he was not crawling as a normal baby and had weakness on his right side. We immediately took him to the doctor, who gave us very bad news. The doctor told us that my son had a stroke while he was in his mother's womb and, as a result, had a hemiparesis (partial paralysis) on the left side of the brain. He was diagnosed with cerebral palsy. The doctor told us that he might not be able to walk and would live as a severely handicapped person. We were completely shocked and devastated to hear the news.

My wife consulted with the radiologist and neurology surgeon at NYU. They had two conflicting opinions. The surgeon advised installing a shunt in the brain to release pressure. The radiology department advised us not to have a shunt as the pressure was, though present once, not there anymore. My wife, as a neurologist, sided with the radiologist and decided not to have the shunt because it might have long-term consequences. Instead, we hired a physical therapist at home, who really did a great job helping my son walk.

We were giving more time to our son. He was very stubborn. His birth name was Ranadeb which he did not like as it is an Indian name. At his insistence, we had to go the Court to change his name to "Roni Dave". Though he was physically handicapped, he was not showing any major deficiency in learning. He resisted any special help from the school. However, he was shy and being teased by his classmates because of his physical condition. We debated on whether to send him to public or private school. In public school he would be treated like others and probably be lost without special attention but might grow up as a stronger person. In private school he would not be overwhelmed by the number of students and would get better attention.

We finally decided to send him to the private school, Lakewood Prep, so that he could have a homey atmosphere. During his early years, we used to take him to Dr. Diamond, pediatric rehabilitation specialist, and Dr. Patel, psychiatrist, at Specialized Children's Hospital, Mountainside, New Jersey, for regular checkups and consultations. Roni was growing as normally as possible, though he could not use his right hand and could not fully support himself on his right leg. At the age of ten,

Roni had surgery on his left knee to keep it straight. However, he was stubborn and finally stopped going to the psychiatrists when he was almost eleven years old. He was having difficulty in reading and comprehending the materials at school. A test detected that because of his hemiparesis he suffers from central auditory processing disorder (CAPD) that affects the way the brain processes auditory information. This affected him getting good grades though he seemed to be an intelligent kid. He was very conscious about his situation. He was depressed inside, and this situation was hard on his mother.

The relationship between Roni and his mother grew apart as my son could not communicate and be close to her, especially when she was suffering from depression. My wife, on the other hand, was very upset as her own son would reject her and not call her "Ma" (mother).

Private Practice

After finishing her residency in neurology at NYU, Rakhi completed her fellowship in EEG/EMG at Rutgers University. She joined a private practice in Staten Island when she declined an offer to join NYU hospital as a junior staff member. After one year she joined a different private practice in Edison, New Jersey. She worked there for two years and was not happy when she was not offered a partnership as promised.

At that point, she decided to start her own private practice in 1994. She immediately got busy and was an attending physician at five hospitals, including JFK, Rahway, South Amboy, Perth Amboy, and Muhlenberg. She moved her office in with my office in Freehold, and after more growth, we moved in 1999 to a five-thousand-square-foot office in Old Bridge.

She tried to hire another doctor to help her. We placed an advertisement in a medical journal and interviewed several doctors. But we did not find the right partner. Finally, Dr. Gupta, a colleague of Rakhi, was interested in quitting his job at the VA Medical Center and joining her private practice. In the end, however, he was concerned about work pressure and declined to join. My wife was very upset about the incident. She really was looking for a helping hand to share the workload.

Finally, she found and hired someone who had just finished her residency program. My wife was initially concerned about this doctor's intention, thinking that she would start her own practice after gaining experience and take patients away. Therefore, Rakhi was hesitant but did hire her. The new doctor was very aggressive, and from the beginning they did not get along well. My wife was showing signs of stress and had to see doctors for a heart problem that was later diagnosed as anxiety attacks. We thought that the aggressive nature of the new doctor might have been a contributing factor to my wife's illness. They were not getting along, and my wife decided to let her go.

Nitech, Inc.

left the AT&T consulting job and joined Timeplex, a subsidiary of Unisys, a computer company, in Woodcliff Lake, New Jersey. It was an hour drive to the office, and I was putting in a lot of hours at work. Finally, I got a transfer and took a supervisory job at the company's new division in Ocean County, which was twenty miles away from our house. This allowed me to spend more time at home. However, it did not last long. When the operation in Ocean County was closed, I had to transfer back to my job in Woodcliff Lake, which I was not happy about.

Finally, when the prototype we were working on in the garage was complete in 1991, I was ready to quit my full-time job and launch the product. At that time I left Timeplex and joined a telecommunication manufacturing company, INC, in Somerset, New Jersey, as a consultant. I was able to convince the management at INC (Dr. Dev Gupta especially) to help build an ISDN interface card for the chassis of their switch product. I got a contract of three hundred thousand dollars, which helped me to hire some people and move to a corporate building in Freehold, New Jersey. We named the company Nitech (New Information Technologies), Inc.

We introduced our first Microsoft Windows (3.0)–based product to the market and sold it to Lucent for ten thousand dollars in 1993. We were making good progress, and our clients, which included AT&T, Lucent, MCI, NASA, Sprint, Nortel, etc., grew exponentially during the first few years. We opened a second sales office in California, with two area sales managers on the East and West Coasts, and we set up sales representatives in all of the major states in America. We then expanded to Europe and Asia. Our annual sales grew to one million dollars. Our staff of about fifty people included full-time and part-time employees. Supporting sales staffs were located all over the USA, Europe, and Asia. I was very excited about the success I was having with the company.

In 2000, I invested about half a million dollars of my personal money to diversify and expand Nitech into the standalone handheld market. We introduced the ADSL test set, a state-of-the-art product primarily targeted for the telephone companies. Our first working prototypes were tried by Italian Telecom and locally by Verizon. I was hoping for big orders from Verizon and other telephone companies and to finally achieve big success.

Nitech got OEM (original equipment manufacturer) offers from companies such as Digital Lightwave, Harris Corporation, and Wandel and Golterman (a German test equipment company) to manufacture and sell exclusively our PC and ADSL products. But unfortunately the economy at the end of 2000 (the last part of President Bill Clinton's second term) was taking a negative turn with the collapse of the Internet boom and the crash of the stock market. This also took a heavy toll on my company's fate. It worsened after the terrorists' attack on the World Trade Center on September 11, 2001.

My Wife's Depression

n 2000, my wife was slowly sliding into depression. We went on vacation to Florida to have some relaxation time, but she did not enjoy it much. She was trying different medicines for depression, such as Zoloft, Prozac, Paxil and Effexor. It became worse, and she fell into a deep depression. She would not go to the hospital and would just lie down in bed for the whole day. She was not eating well and lost weight and looked frail. She would not go to any social event and almost locked herself in the bedroom. I was so concerned that I prayed to God to take her out of this horrific disease. I hoped that she had some other type of ailment that would be more tolerable and treatable.

There is misunderstanding in our society about depression. I was shocked to hear from some of my close friends that they believe depression is not a disease but created by the person because of his or her weak mental state. I took her to a psychiatrist referred by one of Rakhi's best doctor friends. She was reluctant to see any psychiatrist. Usually, a doctor is not a good patient. We initially thought that she was going through post menstruation syndrome (PMS), which causes depression as a result of lack of estrogen. I was surprised to hear from an internist that it is very common that many women who go through this kind of depression never recover fully and become dependent on the drug for the rest of their life. That made me less optimistic about the cure.

She was finally treated by one of her psychiatric colleagues. She tried a different medicine, and it seemed Effexor was finally working. I had difficulty taking care of her while caring for of our partially handicapped son. We had to take him to Children's Specialized Hospital regularly for psychiatrist and therapist appointments.

One fine morning I was thrilled when my wife came to me and said, "I am out of the depression and feeling fine." After two years of being depressed, she was again going to work at the hospitals and her practice. It seemed that she had a second life.

Diagnosis of Parkinson's

When my wife went back to full-time work, she was having pain in her left knee that became intolerable over a short period of time. She got some kind of injection to relieve the pain, but it did not work. She could not sleep because of the excruciating pain and finally decided to have full knee surgery. In November 2002, she had successful knee surgery and went through therapy to regain full control of her leg. She was getting better but showed slowness in her movement. Initially we thought that it was because of her surgery. However, one morning in March of 2003, she told me that she had a tremor in her hand and suspected that she might have Parkinson's disease.

We immediately decided to see Dr. Sudhansu Chokroverty, one of our family friends and a renowned neurologist, under whom Rakhi did her fellowship. He ran a test lasting for about an hour and determined that she was in stage two with Parkinson's disease. We were quite shocked to hear that she who had treated a lot of patients with Parkinson's had the same disease. On the way home, discussing the seriousness of the disease, my wife told me in a calm but confident way that she had a maximum of six to seven years to live in this world.

My wife was very much aware of what she had and would go through in the coming years. Most people, like me, have heard of neurological diseases like Alzheimer's, Parkinson's, MS (multiple sclerosis), and ALS (Lou Gehrig's disease) but are not aware of how devastating this disease could be to the patient and the close family members. Parkinson's is a movement disorder created by the loss of neurons in the brain. It is a degenerative disease and has no cure. Its symptoms are rigidity, stiffness, dyskinesia (involuntary movement), tremors, and loss of balance. I could see in my wife's eyes the seriousness of the disease and, at the same time, some coolness to fight it out. As advised by Dr. Chokroverty the next week I took my wife to see the neurologist Dr. Jacob Sage at UMDNJ for a checkup. My wife had a series of physical tests and was diagnosed with second stage Parkinson's.

We asked ourselves how she got this disease. Initially we thought that she might have symptoms of Parkinson's because of her intake of so many medicines during her illness, which included drugs for treating depression, high blood pressure, sleep disorder, anxiety, and cholesterol. We hoped that the symptoms might be reversible and would go away with time. The doctor later suggested that her depression was an early indication of Parkinson's.

Even today there is no good theory why a person gets Parkinson's. There are two prevailing factors: one is genetic and the other is exposure to chemicals. Rakhi did not belong to either of these two groups, except that she used a lot of chemicals while gardening when she was pregnant. Though some people, like my wife or Michael J. Fox, get Parkinson's at an early age, it is unusual. Like Alzheimer's disease, it usually happens after the age of sixty-five, and the patient can survive with a reasonable quality of life for at least ten to fifteen years with the help of current medicine, which is primarily Sinemet (or seventy-five milligrams of Stalevo, the commercial name).

Parkinson's Disease and Its Symptoms and Treatments

Parkinson's disease (PD) is a brain disorder characterized by the slow degeneration of nerve cells (neurons) in the part of the brain that releases dopamine controlling movement (lack of dopamine). The symptoms of PD appear when over 50 percent of these neurons are no longer functional.

Motor functions affect movement with the following symptoms: tremors, slow movement, rigidity, and difficulty with walking, gait, and balance. As these symptoms become more pronounced, patients may have difficulty walking, talking, or completing other simple tasks. Early symptoms of PD are subtle and occur gradually. In some people the disease progresses more quickly than in others. As the disease progresses, the shaking, or tremor, which affects the majority of PD patients may begin to interfere with daily activities. Other symptoms may include other difficulties such as chewing, and speaking; urinary problems; skin problems. Parkinson's disease is often accompanied by the following additional problems:

•Thinking difficulties. Patient may experience cognitive problems (dementia) and thinking difficulties, which usually occur in the later stages of Parkinson's disease. Such cognitive problems aren't very responsive to medications.

•Depression and emotional changes. People with Parkinson's disease may experience depression. Receiving treatment for depression can make it easier to handle the other challenges of Parkinson's disease.

•Patient may also experience other emotional changes, such as fear, anxiety or loss of motivation. Doctors may give you medications to treat these symptoms.

•Swallowing problems. You may develop difficulties with swallowing as your condition progresses. In typical Parkinson's disease, this is rarely a severe problem. Saliva may accumulate in your mouth due to slowed swallow, leading to drooling.

•Sleep problems and sleep disorders. People with Parkinson's disease often have sleep problems, including waking up frequently throughout the night, waking up early or falling asleep during the day.

•People may also experience rapid eye movement sleep behavior disorder, which involves acting out your dreams. Medications may help your sleep problems.

•Bladder problems. Parkinson's disease may cause bladder problems, including being unable to control urine or having difficulty urinating.

•Constipation. Many people with Parkinson's disease develop constipation, mainly due to a slower digestive tract.

•Patient may feel dizzy or lightheaded when you stand due to a sudden drop in blood pressure (orthostatic hypotension).

•Patient may experience problems with your sense of smell. You may have difficulty identifying certain odors or the difference between odors.

•People with Parkinson's disease lose energy and experience fatigue, and the cause isn't always known.

•People with Parkinson's disease may experience pain, either in specific areas of their bodies or throughout their bodies.

•People with Parkinson's disease may notice a decrease in sexual desire or performance.

Nonmotor functions affect the sensory and autonomic nervous systems and psychological functions. The symptoms of the autonomic nervous system are sweating, bladder problems, low blood pressure when standing up, sexual dysfunction, constipation, and dry skin.

Symptoms of sensory nervous system are numbness, aching, burning, painful cramping, tremors, and back pain. Effects of PD are shifts in mood, agitated and erratic behavior, depression, and dementia. PD is both chronic, meaning it persists over a long period of time, and progressive, meaning its symptoms grow worse over time. Although some people become severely disabled, others experience only minor motor disruptions. Tremor is the major symptom for some patients, while for others tremor is only a minor complaint and other symptoms are more troublesome.

Over one million people suffer from PD in the USA and Canada. The predominant risk factor is age, with few under age fifty, and it rises sharply after the age of sixty-five. Men are more likely to get PD than women.

Environmental toxins used in pesticides and other chemicals may play a role. Industrialized nations have a higher rate of PD. The toxin methyl-phenyl-tetrahydo-pyridine (MPTP) is proved to be directly related to PD. When it is induced in animals (monkeys), they develop PD.

Scientists have linked some genes to PD. Analyses of twins show there may be a genetic link to PD.

PD is diagnosed with the following symptoms: tremor of one or both arms/legs at rest, slow movement, muscular rigidity, and postural instability. Other neurodegenerative disease, metabolic disturbances, or toxins must be ruled out before definitive diagnosis.

Sometimes it takes time to diagnose Parkinson's disease. Doctors may recommend regular follow-up appointments with neurologists trained in movement disorders to evaluate your condition and symptoms over time and diagnose Parkinson's disease.

Parkinson's disease can't be cured, but medications can help control your symptoms, often dramatically. In some later cases, surgery may be advised.

Medications for the early stages of PD are dopamine agonists (Mirapex, Requip, and Permax, etc.). However, the main and only effective medicine for PD is levodopa (Sinemet, Sinemet CR, and Stalevo). Levodopa is converted to dopamine via the action of a naturally occurring enzyme called DOPA decarboxylase. This occurs both in the peripheral circulation and in the central nervous system after levodopa has crossed the blood-brain barrier. Activation of central dopamine receptors improves the symptoms of Parkinson's disease; however, activation of peripheral dopamine receptors causes nausea and vomiting. For this reason levodopa is usually administered in combination with carbidopa, which cannot cross the blood-brain barrier but prevents peripheral conversion of levodopa to dopamine and thereby reduces the unwanted peripheral side effects of levodopa. Use of carbidopa also increases the quantity of levodopa in the bloodstream that is available to enter the brain.

Side effects of PD medications are nausea/vomiting, confusion, drowsiness, dry mouth, dizziness, hallucinations, insomnia, loss of sleep, weight loss (due to loss of appetite) and compulsive behaviors such as hypersexuality, gambling and eating.

In some cases, surgery may be appropriate if the disease doesn't respond to drugs. A therapy called deep brain stimulation (DBS) has now been approved by the U.S. Food and Drug Administration. In DBS, electrodes are implanted into the brain and connected to a small electrical device called a pulse generator that can be externally programmed. DBS can reduce the need for levodopa and related drugs, which in turn decreases the involuntary movements called dyskinesias that are a common side effect of levodopa. It also helps to alleviate fluctuations of symptoms and to reduce tremors, slowness of movements, and gait problems. DBS requires careful programming of the stimulator device in order to work correctly.

Management of PD is a challenge as levodopa complicates the progression of PD. Wearing off of levodopa is managed by changing the dose or adding agents that prolong the duration. Dyskinesia occurs when the levodopa concentration is too high. Lowering the dose and adding a dopamine agonist may be advised.

A patient with PD has to cope with the following difficulties:

1. speech and swallowing problems—eating slowly and choking on food (speech therapy and small bites of food and sips of liquid are recommended)

2. coping with tremors—trouble holding an object (deep brain stimulation surgery has been successful for many PD patients)

3. coping with freezing of motion while walking

4. easing daily tasks, such as cooking, eating, bathing, writing and dressing.

Many changes occur in the brains of people with Parkinson's disease, including:

1. The presence of Lewy bodies. Clumps of specific substances within brain cells are microscopic markers of Parkinson's disease. These are called Lewy bodies, and researchers believe these Lewy bodies hold an important clue to the cause of Parkinson's disease.

2. A-synuclein is found within Lewy bodies. Although many substances are found within Lewy bodies, scientists believe the most important of these is the natural and widespread protein called alpha-synuclein. It's found in all Lewy bodies in a clumped form that cells can't break down. This is currently an important focus among Parkinson's disease researchers.

Risk factors for Parkins on's disease include:

1. Age. Young adults rarely experience Parkinson's disease. It ordinarily begins in middle or late life, and the risk increases with age. People usually develop the disease around age 60 or older.

2. Heredity. Having a close relative with Parkinson's disease increases the chances that you'll develop the disease. However, your risks are still small unless you have many relatives in your family with Parkinson's disease.

3. Sex. Men are more likely to develop Parkinson's disease than are women.

4. Exposure to toxins. Ongoing exposure to herbicides and pesticides may put you at a slightly increased risk of Parkinson's disease.

Certain lifestyle changes as described below may also help make living with Parkinson's disease easier.

1. Healthy eating - A nutritionally balanced diet that contains plenty of fruits, vegetables and whole grains. Eating foods high in fiber and drinking an adequate amount of fluids can help prevent constipation that is common in Parkinson's disease. A balanced diet also provides nutrients, such as omega-3 fatty acids, that may be beneficial for people with Parkinson's disease.

2. Exercise - Exercising may increase your muscle strength, flexibility and balance. Exercise can also improve your well-being and reduce depression or anxiety. Exercises such as walking, swimming, dancing, water aerobics or stretching are also helpful. Exercise with the help of a physical therapist is helpful to avoid any accident such as falls which happen at the later stages of the disease especially because of lack of balance

The following types of alternative medicine may help people with Parkinson's disease:

1. Massage - Massage therapy can reduce muscle tension and promote relaxation. These services, however, are rarely covered by health insurance.

2. Acupuncture - During an acupuncture session, a trained practitioner inserts tiny needles into many specific points on your body, which may reduce your pain.

3. Tai chi - An ancient form of Chinese exercise, tai chi employs slow, flowing motions that may improve flexibility, balance and muscle strength. Tai chi may also prevent falls. Several forms of tai chi are tailored for people of any age or physical condition.

4. Yoga - In yoga, gentle stretching movements and poses may increase your flexibility and balance. You may modify most poses to fit your physical abilities.

5. Meditation - In meditation, you quietly reflect and focus your mind on an idea or image. Meditation may reduce stress and pain and improve your sense of well-being.

6. Music or art therapy - Music or art therapy may help you to relax. Music therapy helps some people with Parkinson's disease to improve their walking and speech. Participating in art therapy, such as painting or ceramics, may improve your fine motor skills and strength and help you express your emotions.

7. Pet therapy. Having a dog or cat may increase your flexibility and movement and improve your emotional health.

Living with any chronic illness can be difficult, and it's normal to feel angry, depressed or discouraged at times. Parkinson's disease presents special problems because it can cause chemical changes in your brain that make you feel anxious or depressed. Parkinson's disease can be profoundly frustrating, as walking, talking and even eating become more difficult and time-consuming.

Although friends and family can be your best allies, the understanding of people who know what you're going through can be especially helpful. For many people with Parkinson's disease and their families, support groups can be good resource for practical information about Parkinson's disease.

To learn about support groups in your community, one may benefit from talking to a mental health professional (psychologist) or social worker trained in working with people with chronic conditions. One also should contact the National Parkinson Foundation or the American Parkinson Disease Association.

Because the cause of Parkinson's is unknown, unfortunately there is no proven ways to prevent the disease. However, some research has shown that caffeine, which is found in coffee, tea and cola, may reduce the risk of developing Parkinson's disease. Green tea also may reduce the risk of developing Parkinson's disease. Some research has shown that regular aerobic exercise may reduce the risk of Parkinson's disease.

Treatment

Dr. Jacob Sage prescribed Mirapex, which is used at the early stage of the treatment, and physical therapy, which is good for making muscles flexible and strong to avoid rigidity. A dopamine agonist is a compound that activates dopamine receptors in the absence of dopamine. Mirapex is a dopamine agonist that activates signaling pathways through the dopamine receptor, ultimately leading to changes in gene transcription. But Rakhi was experiencing the side effect of leg swelling because of Mirapex, which is normal.

We went to see Dr. Cheryl Waters at NYU for a second opinion. She told us that she had done extensive research on Mirapex and promised my wife that she would be normal and even run within a few weeks with the increased dose of Mirapex.

At that time I was planning to take Rakhi to Kolkata, India, for some Ayurvedic (alternative medicine) treatment. This is the first time we went to Kolkata after she had Parkinson's disease. As she was in early stage of her Parkinson's, she did not show any major symptoms of disability, which could upset her family and friends.

Her best friends from her medical college, Sharmistha, Suvra, Anuradha and Snigdha, and friend from high school, Purabi, were very supportive and reassuring. However, when we all made our second trip to Kolkata in December 2006, she was very fragile and could not move at all. They were very upset to see her in this condition for which they inferred her hard and stressful work in her solo practice as a contributing factor. I did not necessarily agree with the remarks but did not get into any arguments. It was a very traumatic experience for all of us. While we were there, we visited renowned neurologist Dr. Dasgupta to get a second opinion. He was referred by Dr. Chokroverty. He did not have any additional advice. I am not much of a believer in Ayurveda medicine, particularly for this type of disease, and when she came back from India, Rakhi could not take the medications as it appeared to conflict with the use of the allopathic medicine that we depended on.

When we came back from India, we went back to see Dr. Cheryl Waters at NYU. She increased the dose of Mirapex, but my wife was not feeling any better.

Trip to the Mayo Clinic

My wife was not running but slowing down rapidly. She suspected she might have Parkinson's plus, i.e., MSA (multiple system atrophy), which is much more severe than typical Parkinson's. As a third opinion, I decided to take her to the Mayo Clinic within a month after we came back from India We rented a room for a week in a hotel across the street from the clinic. She had to go through a series of tests for a couple of days. We had to wait anxiously for the results at the end of the week and were hoping for no MSA. Finally we were ready for the day of the verdict. I accompanied her to the primary physician. She called us into a room and started describing Rakhi's situation.

The results basically reiterated her Parkinson's diagnosis, except they showed that she might have atypical (instead of typical) Parkinson's, which my wife was concerned about to start with. She did not have much of a tremor, which is typical for Parkinson's patients. She was declared as having atypical Parkinson's, also called multiple system atrophy. This is worse than typical Parkinson's because not only are the nerves for movement affected, but so are other surrounding nerves, such as the cerebral nerve, thus compromising balance and speech.

In the current medical science, MSA is less known in terms of treating the disease, and the patient deteriorates faster than those with typical Parkinson's. Life expectancy for a typical Parkinson's patient is anywhere from ten to fifteen years, whereas life expectancy for MSA is five to ten years. My wife was right when she told me once that she had the worse kind of Parkinson's. We came back from Mayo, and Dr. Sage started giving her Sinemet every four hours (four times a day) in addition to Mirapex, as it was not helping.

Quitting the Business

Because of my wife's health condition, we decided to cut our losses and move to smaller offices next to each other, one for Nitech and one for Dr. Guha. During the worst economic condition, Nitech could not survive without any sales from the customers. I was looking for venture money to explore some of the ideas I had with IP phones and high-speed routers/switches. But because of the recession already on the horizon, it was difficult to get money from the venture companies.

I decided to get into the cable TV market. My company became the private cable operator (PCO) of DirectTV and EchoStar and provided integrated voice, video, and Internet data using the Satellite Master Antenna TV (SMATV) system. With this system, one master antenna brought the TV signals into a high-rise building and using a set of receivers and transmitters distributed the signals all over the building through the existing cable. Though initially it looked like an attractive business model, we soon faced stiff competition from the local cable companies, which were regulated and getting special treatment from the local counties.

My wife's practice was affected by her ill health, initially by depression and then by her Parkinson's. She started walking with a cane, and it was risky for her to drive to the office by herself. I started driving her to work. At some point it became risky to continue her practice as she was too weak and unbalanced to perform her duties. I moved all the belongings of Nitech and my wife's business into storage in the basement of our house in July of 2005. It was a sad day for both of us when we both had to quit.

I decided to stay home to take care of her full time. Rakhi used to complain occasionally that she wanted me to be successful in the business (i.e., make money) so that she would not have to work hard and could retire at an early age. I always wanted to work and be successful at the business until I retired at the age of seventy. Nobody thought that it would end this way.

Trip to India for Ayurvedic Treatment

I am spiritual but not so much religious in the traditional sense. My friends suggested that I see some religious gurus and also try alternative medicines, such as kaviraji and homeopathic. I wanted to leave no stone unturned. My brother-in-law in Calcutta, Arup Bose, was very close to his sister and told us about the miracle work of an Ayurvedic doctor in Ahmedabad, India. Rakhi flew to Bombay, where her cousin received her at the airport. From there she flew to Ahmedabad and took a taxi to the office of the Ayurvedic doctor. It was in an alley where the taxi could not go. She decided to go on foot and found that the office was closed until 10:00 a.m.

When she came back, she asked a person holding a dirty cloth when the doctor was coming. He asked my wife whom she was looking for.

She answered, "Doctor."

He replied, "I am the doctor."

She said, "I mean, Doctor—"

He repeated, "I am the doctor."

My wife said, "I came from the USA to see you for my Parkinson's."

The doctor replied that he had been waiting for her. He listened to her case and gave her a couple of bottles of Ayurvedic medicine.

She asked how much she had to pay.

The doctor replied, "Nothing."

She requested that he at least charge some money for the medicine (not necessarily his fee for visit). The doctor said she could pay when she was cured. However, this medicine was not helpful for Rakhi, as its usage conflicted with the use of the allopathic medicine.

Twenty-Fifth Anniversary

We got legally married on December 30, 1980 and were socially married with rituals on January 16, 1981. It was now almost 2006, and our twenty-fifth anniversary would be coming soon. I was not sure how to celebrate it, i.e., whether to invite all of our friends or just celebrate by ourselves. On the one hand, I was not sure whether Rakhi could go through the hassle of a big party or if it would be a good idea to only invite our close friends. I finally decided to do the latter, and a couple of my friends (especially Pushpita and Arati) helped me to make it happen.

It was a grand success. I will remember the event forever. My wife gave speeches about what we were going through in our daily lives. She needed help so that she could stand while giving her speech. I could not help but have tears in my eyes when I gave my speech and talked about my life experience. I was consoled by our friends, and I was glad that I did it.

Daily Chores

My wife used to go to the gym for exercise. Initially I used to drive her to the gym, and I eventually joined to keep her company. She was an early riser. She used to get up at six o'clock, come downstairs, and do her morning exercise while she listened to music, mostly Indian classic music and Rabindra Sangeet (semi-classic). It continued for about a year until she could not walk by herself with a cane. Later I had to help bring her downstairs so that she could continue her daily exercise and listen to music, which is the best companion for a Parkinson's patient.

She was steadily deteriorating. She had to quit going to the gym. She could not walk and was mostly in the wheelchair. At night she went to sleep with the music on. She started taking Stalevo (the commercial name of Sinemet) every three hours, for a total of six times a day. Also, she used to take Ambien to sleep, as she had insomnia (lack of sleep), which is common for Parkinson's patients. But as it was addictive, the doctor prescribed trazodone, which helped her get to sleep and also treated depression and anxiety. In addition, she sometimes took Tylenol PM. She also took Diovan to control her blood pressure.

We finally went to New York for a PET scan to test for positive identification and to determine the degree of severity of the disease. For another opinion, we also went to see Dr. Susan Bressman, chief of neurology at Beth Israel Medical Center, New York, who is an expert in movement disorder. We also wanted to see Dr. Sanderson in Philadelphia, a specialist in treating MSA patients, but we could not meet her as our insurance was not accepted by the practice.

At this point we gave up hope of any miracle medicine. I started doing some research on the Internet. The only hope they were talking about was gene therapy and stem cell research. Both were in the experimental stage and did not provide any solutions at that time. Though stem cell had promise, our then president, Mr. George W. Bush, made the research work impossible because of his personal religious beliefs.

Trip to Brazil

One of our doctor friends mentioned the healing person in Abadiania, Brazil, John of God. I looked on the Internet and was impressed by what I saw. I immediately booked the tickets and reserved the hotel. I packed up our suitcases, and we went to the capital of Brazil. We had to take the connecting flight from another airport. We missed the bus that would take us to the other airport, so we decided to take a taxi. The cars were bumper to bumper. The traffic was so bad (worse than what I have seen in Calcutta), that by the time we arrived at the airport, we missed the flight and were booked on a later flight.

When we arrived at the ashram, which was more than an hour's drive from the airport, we were tired and ready to go to bed. The next morning when we were having breakfast, I sat near a lady, Susan, who came from California and had hepatitis C. She was told by her doctor that her days were numbered. From then on while at the ashram, we got together every morning at breakfast. She is one of the nicest persons I have met in my life. Since then she has been a good friend of mine, and I still keep in touch with her and discuss about spiritual matters on a regular basis.

John of God's patients typically stay at Abadiania for two weeks, but they can live there for as long as they want. For those who believe, John of God is a sixty-nine-year-old miracle man and spiritual medium. He is a man with no medical degree and little formal education. Yet the healer performs surgeries in an effort to help the sick and dying. John of God grabs what looks like a kitchen knife from a silver tray and appears to scrape it over the right eye of a believer. He then wipes a viscous substance from the blade onto the patient's shirt. John of God says, "I am not the one curing those who come to me. It's God who heals. I am just the instrument." According to him, while his body is taken over by the spirits, he conducts the raw surgeries without using appropriate and sterilized devices that are difficult to observe.

I have to say that my wife did not get any apparent benefit by seeing John of God and my friend, Susan, though visited the place several times, still have problem with her lever. However, somebody else might have different and positive experiences because of their strong faith and believe.

Trip to Alaska

I became close to a number of families during my life in the USA. Soon after I arrived, when I lived in Randolph in northern New Jersey, I was one of the founding members of a community center called ICC. During that time I became close to two men, Mr. Dutta and Mr. Dhar. They were older than me. It seems that I always make friendships more easily with older people. We used to take vacations together and visit at least once a year.

Mrs. Dutta became seriously ill with a viral disease that could be fatal. With proper care and medicine, she recovered and gained weight with a heavy dose of a steroid. One morning Mrs. Dhar found a lump in her breast and went to see the doctor. She was immediately tested and diagnosed with breast cancer. She had some early success with radiation and chemo therapy and decided not to have a mastectomy.

I still vividly remember the evening at our house when Mr. Dutta, Mr. Dhar, and I discussed the fates of our wives, who were going through their difficult health experiences. Mrs. Dhar's cancer relapsed after a couple of years, and she died within a few months.

Rakhi and I decided to take a cruise to Alaska. I thought it would be a good idea for Rakhi to stay in one place without much movement and, at the same time, enjoy lots of food and musical performances at night, both of which she loved very much. We decided to take Mr. Dhar with us. One of my family friends, Mrs. Chatterjee, also came. It was a grand seven-day journey we will never forget. We took a train trip inland. My wife started writing a poem about Krishna Dhar.

We also took a helicopter trip to the glacier. Rakhi was not able to walk and therefore had to sit with an attendant while the rest of us hiked to a higher altitude. She later old me that she had a pleasant time with the attendant and wrote a poem about the experience.

Taking Care of My Wife

As I mentioned, I had decided to leave my business to take care of my wife full time. In the beginning, through an agent I hired a caregiver who happened to be a Philippine lady. We were moderately happy with her. I had to pick her up on Monday morning from her home in Edison and give her a ride back on Friday evening. She used to stay with us during the work week. She left us after about six months, as she had to travel to the Philippines to see her family members.

I then hired an Indian (Gujrati) caregiver, Mrs. Patel, who used to live in the neighboring town. She was also a caring lady. However, my wife used to get into arguments with her sometimes. A person with Perkinson's shows rigidity and gets irritated and angry easily as they have to depend on others most of the times and get into arguments easily when they are not heard or responded immediately. She finally left us after almost a year, at which point I found another Philippine caregiver, who was also very caring. My wife became very close to her over time. She also used to stay with us during the week but had to go back to her home in Staten Island for the weekend.

She eventually left as she wanted to spend more time with her boyfriend. At that point, I hired her friend, another Philippine lady, with whom my wife got into arguments occasionally. We had to let her go after six months.

As it was difficult to get a dependable and caring caregiver, at the beginning of 2007, I decided to take a certified training course in home health aid (HHA) so that I was capable of taking care of my wife in case I had any problem finding a full-time caregiver available to live seven days a week with us.

Finally I hired a caregiver, Pushpa, from Sri Lanka, whom I had found through a newspaper's advertisement. She happened to be the best among all the caregivers I had hired. She was very caring and understandable about my wife's situation. She knew how to handle the situation and avoid getting into arguments with Rakhi. Though she was not a good cook or housecleaner, she always kept Rakhi company and took care of her. Over time she became a member of our family.

My wife was gradually losing her voice. In the early stages of the disease, she used to have conversations with some of her close friends, but these days she could not have a long conversation over the phone. This was difficult for her and her friends, so she would just have to talk briefly on the phone. Mostly, her friends visited her at home, and occasionally I used to take her to their houses. However, it was more and more difficult because of

Rakhi's lack of mobility. For a while, I tried to keep her engaged with the company of friends.

The things she most enjoyed were listening to music and reading books. Though she was quite alert, and her memory was very strong, I noticed sometimes she was not reading but only holding the book, pretending to read as she could not concentrate because of Parkinson's.

At the beginning, I had no problem understanding what she was saying. But it gradually became more and more difficult to understand her.

She was also so fragile that she had to stop the yoga lessons with the guidance of her teacher, Mr. Singh, whom we hired on an hourly basis to come to our home three days a week.

This was the most difficult time we were going through. We were losing her at a rapid rate. She started to lose control of her bowels and bladder and had to wear adult diapers for a long time, which I had to put on her and clean up with my own hands. I used to give her a bath and feed her. Though she could eat most of the time, she had to be fed sometimes, depending on her condition.

She used to take Stalevo seven times a day (every two and a half hours), from 6:00 a.m., when she woke up, to 11:00 p.m., when she went to bed. Luckily, Stalevo, which was the miracle medicine for typical Parkinson's patients, also worked for her as an atypical patient. She went through a cycle of being in an on state and then an off state. An on state means when the medication is working and symptoms are controlled and an off state means when the effect of medicine wears off and goes back to a state of decreased mobility. When she started going down, she would take the medicine and then come up within half an hour and would stay for about one hour before she would go down again.

The Parkinson's patients have chance of losing weight especially at the later stage when they lose their appetite and interest in food partly because they cannot swallow and find eating a challenging task. Therefore, it is very important for a Parkinson's patient to consult with the doctor so that they have a well-balanced, nutritious diet with enough calories to maintain weight, which should include high-fiber foods such as vegetables, cooked dried peas and beans, whole-grain foods, bran, cereals, pasta, rice, and fresh fruit. At the end, she could not take solid food anymore (only mashed or liquid food). She started losing weight as she was not eating properly. At this point it was OK to lose weight as she had been slightly on the heavy side. But I was concerned about the rate at which she was losing weight. She was not getting enough protein. I started cooking liquid food, such as mashed potatoes and Progresso soup and giving her Ensure.

I was worried one day when I noticed skin had come off from her buttocks This was serious and alarming and could have been fatal. I immediately asked for a visiting nurse.

The nurse said that it was not a major problem and gave us patches to use, which helped her skin to heal.

Also, she was having pain in her left shoulder. I took her to see an orthopedic doctor, who found no major problem but advised physical therapy.

I could not think of sending her to a nursing home. I wanted to keep her at home as long as I could take care of her by myself. I did not want to think of the worst day in my life when I would not be able to take care of the situation and would have to send her to a nursing home. I was afraid of the inevitable day when I would have to give her tube feedings, which I was trying to delay because it would restrict her mobility and hamper her moral strength. She was having problems with swallowing and was advised not to eat solid food but only liquid food. One good thing was that she was not depressed (though she had severe depression at one time) and was mentally strong.

Our Daughter, a Doctor

Our daughter, Koel, was doing very well at school and finally got into a combined (six-year) medical program at Jefferson Medical College after finishing two years at Penn State. My wife started showing signs of depression when Koel left home for her undergraduate degree at Penn State. Koel did not have to face and experience the difficult time we were experiencing with Rakhi. When she came home on holidays, she spent most of the time with her school friends and little time at home. It seemed that she did not want to face the difficulty her mother was going through. She was very busy and under a lot of pressure at medical school. She kept herself more and more distant from us, especially her mother.

When Koel was in Philadelphia at Jefferson Medical School, we used to meet her for dinner on a regular basis. She finished her MD degree with honors and went to Northwestern Children's Hospital in Chicago for a residency in pediatrics. When she moved to Chicago for residency, we would not talk to her for months. I thought we were losing her. When she would come home on holidays, she avoided spending time with her mother. It seemed that she could not face Rakhi's health situation. She did not want to take my advice to go for a fellowship. Instead she started her first job at Princeton Medical Center in New Jersey so that she could stay near home. When we discovered she was coming back to New Jersey, we were glad that we would be able to see and spend more time with her. Also, I noticed that she was thinking about marriage, as her close friends were getting married. But she ruled out any advice from our side on this matter.

Roni, our son, was finally graduating high school. Initially I thought I would be happy if he got admission to Rutgers or NJIT for his undergraduate program. Because of his seizure problem, he was not willing to go to college outside New Jersey. Also, he insisted on living at home while attending college. Because of his situation, I finally decided to send him to Brookdale Community College, which was five miles from our home. He would be able to study and get a degree from Rutgers University in business with a "communiveristy" program. I invited some close friends and celebrated his graduation with a party.

Deteriorating Faster

Because of the atypical nature of the disease (Parkinson's plus), Rakhi was deteriorating faster than a typical patient. For a typical patient, one could live quite long (about fifteen years). An atypical patient could expect to live about ten years, depending on the severity. However, it was difficult to predict how fast any patient would deteriorate. One day Rakhi seemed to be doing well, and another day she was not well. I got scared. Though she had not faced additional difficulties in regard to swallowing, she was eating poorly and losing weight.

At the end she could not take a bath by herself and could not sit down in a chair on her own (usually she slipped away from the chair). She still loved ice cream but could not feed herself. We still tried to have her go up and down our staircase to maintain some exercise, but she had to be held so that she did not fall. She stayed mostly quiet, not talking much, as she either could not talk or could not be understood. This was particularly tragic, as she was quite alert mentally. She did not look at people, kept her head down, and tried to keep herself busy doing something (most of the time cleaning her surroundings). The most tragic part was that she was mentally alert and strong and showed no depression. She could even remember days from her childhood. As she had less energy, the doctor increased the dose of Stalevo to 150 mg, and, as a result, her level of energy increased.

Last Few Months

Rakhi lost so much weight that she could not be recognized at the end. She did not smile and communicate with friends as she used to when they came to visit and keep her company. She did not even look at them but turned the other way. I should also mention couple of new habits she had, which cannot be explained. She would pick up dirt from the table where she was sitting by. She also had a tendency to try to pull on a shirt or curtain and play with it. She kept silent most of the time and only said "yes" or "no." She would give us a slight smile once in a while to make her presence known. I knew that her memory was strong and she understood everything taking place around her. However, it was difficult to fathom what she was thinking to herself when she could not talk.

On a typical day, I woke her up at 7:30 a.m. and administered her first medicine (125 mg Stalevo) and then got our son, Roni, ready for school. I moved her to her side to go to sleep for another hour in the bed. After Roni went to school, I brought the breakfast (croissant, egg, milk, cookie, and a sweet). This was one of the main meals of the day and why I wanted to make sure she ate it all. After about one hour, when she was done, I called the caregiver to take her downstairs to give her bath, at about 11:00 a.m.

She enjoyed her bath every day and was given lunch (rice and fish) at about 1:00 p.m. Because of the swallowing problem, it was difficult for her to eat. Most days she only ate one meal, either lunch or dinner. After lunch, she went upstairs to watch TV with the caregiver, at about 3:00 p.m. She was given tea sometimes at 5:00 p.m. She came downstairs at 8:00 p.m. for her dinner. She was a slow eater those days. She finished her dinner with ice cream and went to bed, at about 11:00 p.m. I fed her milk in bed before she went to sleep, at midnight. I wondered sometimes about what she thought about her life, as she did not talk too much those days.

It was terrifying to fathom what would happen to a patient in her situation at the end, which I came to know through the knowledge she shared with me and the studies I did using the Internet. The patients in her situation die not because of the disease but of the complications caused by the disease, e.g., pneumonia, bedsores, heart failure, or from weakness.

I have to mention that the patient goes through the most difficult time mentally and physically. Also, the family members who take care of the patient on a daily basis get seriously affected mentally. They have to be strong mentally and physically and make sure that they do not get burnt out.

Losing a person dear to you is so tragic that it cannot be explained to others. It is heartbreaking when you lose someone suddenly or over a short period of time as a result of an accident or a disease such as cancer. It is more devastating when you lose a person over a long period who (once full of life, vigor, and energy) deteriorates gradually and ultimately to a zombie (zero) state with almost no ability or function. Witnessing this cannot be explained in words.

Last Days

Pushpa, Rakhi's caregiver, used to go to New York to visit her brother once in a while. On the evening of July 21, a Tuesday, she went to New York and planned to come back the next night. In the past, she would come back a couple of days later than she was supposed to. This time I reminded her not to take an extra day, as I was not feeling good about Rakhi getting along without her.

Wednesday morning, as usual, I woke Rakhi up at 7:30 a.m. and administered her first medicine (125 mg Stalevo). Later, I brought the breakfast (croissant, egg, milk, cookie, and a sweet) and fed her well. Around eleven o'clock, when she was done, I took her downstairs to give her bath. She enjoyed her bath, and I took her to the sun-room to lie down.

At about 1:00 p.m., I brought a fish sandwich from Wawa, and we ate together. Later, she had some fruit while she was lying down on the bed and watching TV. I was also watching TV and keeping her company. In the evening, I cooked chicken and mixed vegetables. She ate so well, which made me very happy. After dinner she had ice cream and went to bed at about 11:00 p.m. I was sleeping beside her and listening to the Rabindra Sangeet. I comforted her by softly touching her forehead and hair. I knew from the past that she enjoyed when I did this.

The next morning I woke up and followed the same routine. As usual Pushpa did not show up either in the evening or the next morning though she had promised. After giving Rakhi breakfast, I took her downstairs to give her bath. She enjoyed her bath, and I lay her down in the sun-room as I did the day before.

At about 1:00 p.m., I again went to Wawa and bought a tuna fish sandwich, and Rakhi and I ate together. Later, as she wanted, we shared some fruit. I then let her lie down on the bed so that she could watch TV. These days she had a tendency to try to pull on a shirt or curtain and play with it. She was trying to sleep on her side while reaching and pulling the curtain. I told her not to do that but to watch TV.

It was about 2:00 p.m. My son was watching TV in the next room. After using the computer upstairs, my daughter had to go out to see her friend. After my daughter left, I went upstairs to check my e-mail. After a few minutes, when I came downstairs to see my wife, I saw her lying on her side with her face down on the pillow. I rolled her over and saw she was not breathing and her face was a little bluish. I tried to give CPR to resuscitate her. But when I could not do it successfully, I was frantic and called 911 immediately, at about 3:00 p.m. They came within about fifteen minutes. They also tried to resuscitate her but could not. They then took her in the ambulance to the nearest hospital, where she was pronounced dead.

I realized that I had lost my best friend. Pushpa called me from the train in the evening and told me that she was coming back. I told her that Rakhi was not with us anymore.

Rakhi as a Person

Rakhi always had a keen interest in the arts and was involved in cultural activities with the Indian Community Center (ICC) from its inception. Rakhi also played an active role in several other Bengali organizations: she was president of NJPA in 1994 and a life member of Kallol and Ananda Mandir. Because of her natural creative talents and strong artistic inclination, Rakhi was often given the responsibility of decorating the puja temple.

It was hard to watch Rakhi the last few years. I remember Rakhi when she was handling many things at the same time. She was blessed with so many talents. She was a dedicated physician, passionate artist, painter, sculptor, writer, and selfless wife and mother. Most importantly, she was beautiful outside and inside. Whatever she did, she did for others, not for herself. I was lucky to have a wife with so many qualities. We will miss her greatly and always cherish the memories of her time here with us.

At the same time, she was not perfect and had some shortcomings like any other human being. She was pessimistic, not content with what she had, and she could not find peace within herself. She was stubborn, outspoken, undiplomatic, ambitious, and showed less interest and skill in dealing with household matters. She was so busy in her profession that she did not have much time for her family members, including children and husband. She spent her spare time with her friends, talking on the phone or accompanying them to religious activities and places (such as temples). In hindsight, I feel she could have managed her professional obligations more efficiently so that she could have spent more time with the family.

Ultimately, like other Parkinson's patients she treated for so many years, Rakhi could not escape the fate that was bestowed upon her by a higher power. After undergoing knee surgery in 2003 at the age of fifty, Rakhi diagnosed herself with Parkinson's. Unfortunately, she had a very progressive and severe form of the disease known as atypical Parkinson's (a.k.a Parkinson's plus). Though the disease greatly affected her balance and mobility, she continued to practice up until the spring of 2005. During this period, Rakhi spent much of her spare time painting and sculpting, creating beautiful pieces of art. She always enjoyed and excelled at painting but did not have the time to pursue her talent earlier in life due to her demanding professional career.

Some Memorable Moments

Though Rakhi and I had a difficult life during her last 10 years while she was suffering from severe kind of Parkindson's followed by severe depression, we had some memorable moments, recollection of which still help me today to live on.

When she got out of depression, she came back to the same person with smile in her face, who was always active with something such as painting, music, and writing besides her busy professional work. The paintings she made during her illness were unforgettable and priceless. I remember those days when she used to get up early in the morning, go down stairs to the living room, turn on the CD player and do exercise while listening to the music. When she could not move, I used to help her to go down stairs. It was sad to see her in this situation but made me proud of my wife to watch that she would not surrender to the disease.

I heard a story from one of my friend later who once visited my wife because of her seizure problem. She told my wife, "I am worried what will happen to me and my family". My wife responded, "Look at me. I am at much worse shape than you are". What will you do if you are in my situation? You have to fight it out".

It was nice to hear another story from another friend, Sebika, who was discussing with my wife about her situation and future plan at her early stage of her Parkinson's. She said, "I talked to my husband. I feel good. My husband said she will take care of me".

My wife liked dancing during parties. On one occasion while we were attending a wedding ceremony, she decided to get up, start dancing and fell down as she lacked balance because of her Parkinson's. Some of our friends were understandably broken and distressed in front of her while she was consoling them. I will never forget this incident which showed her strength and capacity under the extreme situation.

My wife used to tell me at her last stage, "My only worries are what will happen to my son when I am gone." I used to tell her, "Do not worry; I will make sure he is ok."

Looking Back at My Life

My life as an immigrant has been eventful. I had to work hard to prove and establish myself in all aspects of life. After marriage, we tried to build a better life together for all of us and faced and shared all kinds of difficulties and challenges along the way. The challenges were compounded by the fact that we had to pay a lot of attention to the children to make sure they were raised properly, especially because of my son's health situation.

Rakhi and I were both ambitious and became busy with our professional lives in addition to taking care of our children. Once in a while, we got into silly arguments, mostly without good reasons. If I could change something, I would change our life style to have less ambition, not spending so much time running around. We could have had less tension and stress and have spent more time together ourselves and also with the children, which is very important to keep one's marriage healthy. We should have treated each other more often on special occasions, like birthdays and Mother's and Father's Days. I am a passionate and romantic person. Sometimes

I expected a simple "thanks" from Rakhi, which was hard to come by.

When Rakhi and I first found out about her Parkinson's disease, that first night lying down in our bed, we held hands together, and I promised my unconditional love and support. Rakhi and I fought the disease to the end the best we could. She never complained about her difficulties, and she took on the challenges with a smile. I cannot think of anybody else who could handle the worst situation in a more courageous, graceful, and dignified way than she did.

Politics and Religion

would be remiss to write this book and not talk about some political, religious, and spiritual aspect of our lives.

There are some important issues in our lives on which we take the extreme position, either on the left or on the right, based on our political and religious beliefs. For religious reasons, there is a tendency to deny the research of embryonic stem cell research, which is the only hope for all kinds of diseases, including nerve degenerative disease. The argument is we should not kill the eggs that could be used to produce life. In this case the embryonic eggs are sitting frozen in a tube forever and are not claimed by anybody and will never be used for creating a life. These cells are embryonic, which can grow to become a human body. They can be converted to a cell of any part of the body, such as brain cells to replace dying cells for Alzheimer's or Parkinson's' patients. As there is undoubtedly an ethical issue, it is understandable that we have to be careful about how we use these embryonic cells. But it does not make sense that we should watch close relatives dying in front of us because we are trying to protect the rights of the unborn. We are misplacing importance by giving equal rights to the born and the unborn. But we have no problem ignoring the millions of people who are dying. It just does not make sense.

Self-Realization

We are born in a society where we do not have control of all matters and our final destiny. However, I strongly believe we are makers of our fortune for the most part. Our intelligence, environment, and education can give us an edge. But, we are primarily responsible for how we lead our lives, how we act (deeds), what judgments we make, and what we achieve as a result.

However, success has a different meaning for different people. There is no doubt that money plays a very important role in life. But money does not take us anywhere if peace is not there. It is important to know ourselves and what we want in life. Whatever situation (good or bad) we are in, we have to be optimistic, make best out of the current situation and find contentment and peace within ourselves. Let us try to see the glass half full instead of half empty. There is nothing wrong with working hard to achieve higher goals, but let us be always happy with what we have. Let us love ourselves. If we cannot love ourselves, we cannot love others. Also, have some good friends to share joys and sorrows in our life. There is one life to live. We should love the persons dear to us and around us.

The other important factor is health. When we are young, we work hard and do not think about our mortality. When we reach fifty, we experience different kinds of health issues depending on genes and lifestyles, including diet and exercise. Sometimes I wonder how my wife developed this disease. She did not conform to any of the two most prevailing theories of having Parkinson's. Her family did not have this disease, and she was not exposed to any chemicals. However, she was not good at handling stress and tension. She had periods of anxiety and depression occasionally, which might have contributed to her Parkinson's, though there is no scientific data supporting this.

We are always tested, especially in bad times. Our successes or achievements are not measured by how much money we have but how we handle our difficult and challenging situations with strength and courage. We may wonder why we have more challenges and difficulties than others. God is always testing us, and maybe there is a greater purpose for us having the problem. Perhaps one is the right person to handle it, through which one can achieve enlightenment toward nirvana. To achieve the best outcome, we should not be afraid of death but face and do our karma (deed) to our greatest ability with strength, honor, love, and compassion.

I feel fortunate, blessed, and privileged that I had the opportunity to love my wife from the bottom of my heart and take care of her with unconditional love and give all I had, especially when she needed it. As a result, I find that I have become a better person and feel peace within myself. This is my salvation. I feel deeply that I was placed in this world to serve my wife. She was my soul mate.

Conclusion

With great sadness and difficulties, I came to the realization that Dr. Chandralekha Guha (Rakhi, as we affectionately called her) left us forever to continue her journey to a better place.

Rakhi and I both had our share of challenges and difficulties in our lives. But God showed both of us how to handle the challenges in the worst moments of life with dignity, courage, and strength. She was always full of life and never complained about her situation. She could not talk at the end but let her presence be known with a simple smile.

We were lucky to have each other. During the last ten years of her life, it was extremely difficult to watch her going through drastic physical changes. Rakhi was once hardworking, vibrant, and energetic. But at the end, she could not walk, speak, or eat and looked frail and lost a lot of weight. Rakhi was an established neurologist. It is kind of sad that she treated patients with the same disease she had.

Relationships are not built in one day. Over time and through the long journey we took, our relationship was built with unconditional love and without any expectations.

The death of a loved one is the worst thing that can happen to anyone. I survive day by day, and the loneliness sometimes overwhelms me. Time is really not the healer. We never move on.

Rakhi is survived by her loving husband (Dilip), daughter (Koel), son (Roni), and her elder sister (Chitralekha Pal) who has resided in Los Angeles, California, for the last forty years. Rakhi's legacy lives on through her children. Roni will start college this fall, and Koel is working as a pediatrician in Princeton, New Jersey.

Chandralekha (Rakhi) was born in Kolkata, India.
Though she has not had formal training,
she began painting when she was a teen.

During Rakhi's 15 year medical profession
she rarely found time to paint and write.
The writings, paintings, and sculptures depicted here
represent some of her works mostly in 2000,
before her diagnosis of parkinson's
and MSA (Multiple System atrophy).

Due to her symptoms, Rakhi was unable
to paint or write after 2005.

A Tale of the City

By Rakhi Guha

I went to visit Calcutta last year. I was planning to go to Puri from there. I booked a ticket in advance to reserve a berth in Jagannath Express. Today was Saraswati Puja for Hindus as well as Eid festival for Muslim. Though I started one and a half hour earlier and our car zoomed through the Garia Bypass, I was late by five minutes and watched the train leaving the train platform in front of me. My childhood friend, Purabi, came to the station to see me off. "When Jagannath has called me, I must go to Puri", said to Purabi.

Puri Express is going to leave within few hours. I bought a ticket at higher price after waiting at the long line. Purabi was very much opposed to the idea. "I will not let you go without the reserved seat", said Purabi. "It is so crowded that you have no choice but to hang on to the window. You may fall down", said Purabi.

I was waiting on the seventh line to board the train. Suddenly I heard that a party with a bridegroom was also going to Puri and an extra bogie had been added to the train for them. The person who was selling the ticket said to me," You also get on this bogie. It should fit another extra person." I followed his instruction. As soon as I boarded the train, I fell asleep and woke up when the train reached Bhubaneswar station where the bridegroom party deboarded the train. I was the only person in the compartment. The ticket collector boarded our compartment. He started talking about good days and bad days of his family during the rest of the journey. Finally I reached the Puri station to see Jagannath. I felt that this kind of pleasant meeting with such ordinary people with good hearts is possible only in India.

Road to Agra

By Rakhi Guha

Several years ago, my family and I went to India on a vacation. On our way back to the States we decided to visit Delhi, Agra and Jaipur. We hired a car from Delhi to Agra. We passed a number of mosques. During midday, call of "Ajah" boomed from their microphone – "Allah Ho Akbar"

There was a blockade on the road in front of us. The driver had to back the car. To alert the passersby, his car stereo started playing "Jay Jagadisha Hare…". Just at that moment, my rental cell phone started ringing. The ring tone played – "Sare Jahanse Achha, Hindustan Hamara, Sare Jahanse Achha". The call was coming from America.

The three sounds of Allah, Jagadishwar and Hindustan made the amazing, strangest symphony I have ever heard. Unity is Diversity!

Snow in the Summer

By Rakhi Guha

(Dr. Rakhi Guha, wrote this poem
during her trip to Alaska in 2005.)

Snow in the summer? Is it possible?"
Yes, I saw it in the heaven, quite possible.

The top of the mountain is covered with ice
While walking there, I fell down twice
Finally I grabbed a chair
To enjoy the beauty and the fresh air
The guy half of my age sat next to me
and said, together with you,
I like to enjoy the beauty.
He asked me about my daughter, of course
She is busy 'cause she is the medical school.
Next year in her graduation I will give her my
white coat and stetho.
The guy said, "That will be cool"

He will go to University of Utah to study English
Major
I said that will be hard as you have to read
Shakespeare
Then the guy stood up and said
"It has been very nice talking to you".
I said the same and congratulation to you".
"When you graduate with English major
Your first poem will be "Snow in the Summer".

"ব্রাজিলের পথে"

রাখী গুহ

চলো যাই ব্রাজিলেতে, দু পাশে কালো মাঠ,
  মাঝখানে রাস্তা কাটা ।
সকালবেলা উঠে দেখি, এতো কালো মাঠ নয়,
  এ যে উপত্যকা ।
সারি সারি পাহাড়গুলো নেমে গেছে নীচে,
সে এক অপরূপ শোভা, বলি কী আর মিছে ।
অচেনা মুখ, অচেনা হাত বাড়ায় আমারদিকে,
"আন্টি, তুমি কেমন আছ?", মিষ্টি সুরে ডাকে ।
সঙ্গে আছে আর এক যুবক, শুনেছি তার ভাই,
মাখায় হয়েছে lymphoma, এখানে এসেছে তাই ।
এ রোগ কি আর সহজে সারে ?
মনে পড়ে সেই পুরোন সুর –
"বিশ্বাসে মিলায় বস্তু, তর্কে বহুদুর" ।

91

On way to Brazil

(Neurologist Dr. Rakhi Guha, a patient of Parkison's Plus disease, visited a Brazilian spiritual hermitage for treatment in alternative medicine. The poem in the previous page was written during her visit to Brazil and, retaining the original thought, translated from Bengali by Sushmita Dutta)

Come, let's go to Brazil
Roads curved through uphill
Blending into black meadows
With endless, footsteps
Unknown faces, untold tales
Seeking helping arms in hopes,
Roads curved through black meadows
Beneath uphill, let's go to Brazil.

Lights of dawn unveiled
A serene beauty, improbable.
The black meadows visible
As upland, plateau
Edged in mountain rows

Astounding, amazing, when
An unknown face extended
A nameless hand and said,
"How are you aunty"?
Another young lad with him
I believe was his brother, stood apart
Infected by Lymphoma in the head
So, he was at the hermitage.
Does this disease get cured? Quickly?
I asked. Well, faith can cure for sure
Or maybe who knows? Distrust delivers distrust
Irredeemable hopelessness. So, faith matters.
Thus, faith remains.

Ananda Mandir

By Rakhi Guha

Mother First I bow down to your feet
In this Ananda Mandir, as we say it,
Let us all come with a holy spirit;
Let us here het together
We all come to you 'Mother'
Who has what and who knows what
All these things stay away from here
We only come to you with our holy spirit here

By uttering mantra and worshiping Devi
That is not end of the day
Decorating Devi with our local talents
And cooking Kichuri make us happy and gay

If we stay away from here
We stay away from you farther
Let us forget all the division and let us sing
Vivekananda's message ad Martin luther King

Taking Care of my wife Rakhi with Parkinson's

Don't forget the poor Indian;
They are your brother
Don't forget the Harijans & lower caste;
They are your brother, your bloods.

"অনুপকে"

রাখী গুহ

(Rakhi wrote this poem for Anup, a
family friend, for his 40th birthday.)

আজ সেদিনের কথা খুব মনে পড়ে,
বাইরে টাপুর টুপুর বৃষ্টি পরে।
"রাখীদি, ছাতাটা একটু শেয়ার করুন।
মনে মনে ভাবলাম, ঠিক চিনলাম না তো কে এই তরুণ?
বেশতো দেখতে সুপুরুশটি,
চুলে আবার তেরীকাটা, বেশভূষায় পরিপাটি।
আমেরিকায় এসেছিলে মনে নিয়ে আশা
যে ভাল হয়ে যাব, এই দৃঢ় বিশ্বাস।
কিন্তু ডাক্তার ত দিল না কোন আশ্বাস।
বললে আর বেশী দেরী নেই, মাএ ছ মাস,
এরকম ছ মাস ছ মাস করে গেল কত ছয় মাস।
তবু আমেরিকায় থাকার মিটলা না বাস,
আমিওত একদিন আমেরিকায় এসেছিলাম
মনে কত নিয়ে আশা,
এদেশটা luxury চূড়ান্ত, তার নেই ভাষা।
ভেবেছিলাম ডাক্তারি করব, হব লাখপতি।
সবই কপালের লিখন নাহলে এ গতি?
But miracle happens with faith in God
If it happens to them,

it will happen to my son and me
Have a happy 40th birthday and
many happy returns of the day
Finally I like to say to you that as long as you live,
enjoy each and every day.

আশার আলো

রাখী গুহ

নিস্তব্ধ রাত, শুধু ঘড়ির টিকটিক আওয়াজ
খুব লিখতে ইচ্ছে করে, কী লিখি আজ?
নিজের মনের কথা, মনেতেই থাক না
আজকে লিখব যত জীবনের ভাবনা।

কত আশা করে এসেছিনু এ দেশে
জীবনের মোড়টা কোথা ঘুরে গেল এসে,
আজ, দেহ বড় শক্ত লাগে, যেন তাসের দেশে
কত যে শক্তি, কতই সাহস কী হয়ে গেল শেষে

তাইতো আজ মাকে ডাকি, মাগো শোনো আমার কথা।
দাওগো শক্তি, দাও সামর্থ্য, তোমার চরণে করি মাথা
একদিন ভোরবেলা উঠে যেন দেখি
শরীরটা হালকা হয়েছে, সহজে চলছি, একি ?
তবু কিছু পেয়েছি জীবনে, যা পাইনি আগে
ভোরের সূর্যোদয়, আকাশে কী শোভা জাগে
আর পূর্ণিমার চাঁদের আলো। মনে কত লাগে ভাল
শরতের বাতাসে দোলা কাশ ফুলগুলি,
প্রকৃতি হাসিয়া দেয়, চোখে তারে তুলি।

সময় ছিল না এ দৃশ্য দেখার
আমের মোহে মত হয়ে, কজে কদাকার।
আজ আমি শান্ত, আমার চিত অতি স্হির
জীবনটা যেন এক শান্তির নীড়।

Light of Hopes

(English adaptation of the poem in the
previous page by Sushmita Dutt)

Silent night, watertight
clock ticking, beating light
I want to write….yes,
I want to write, but
write what?
Can't those whispering,
slurring heart's content
remain in heart, for now?
Un-spoken, un-heard?

What's the rush? I said,
calm down, see the frown
on life's face coated with
dust from the past, so,
I have to write. Yes,
I will have to write.
Touch life, write on

Un-read worries, fears
apprehensions, tears.
Touch life, so close
  that I can feel it.
Write on it. Tear it apart.

Life. Listen, I had come
To this land of
untouched places
nameless faces
Unknown feelings
and consigned hopes.

Life. You took your turn
for reasons unknown
and, my body became stiff.
As if, my flesh and bones

had hardened in fear
to caution that
I had lost my strength in vain.

Lord! Have mercy! Please.
Give back my strength
Touch me. Caress me.
Your touch is the only touch
Divine. Makes me breathe
Feel that I am living.

Have mercy. Lord,
have mercy, Please.

And then, one morning,
I woke-up feeling
Light, easy and lively.
As if something attained
that was un attained…

The rising sun dawning
moonlit stars glowing
autumn winds blowing
grass glowers dancing…
My God, I never glanced
outside my window
to be so close to life, and
now, look at me, I am calm
I am cheered, life is zestful
life is peaceful like a nest,
My loving nest, at last.

"মাকে"

রাখী গুহ

আবার সেই নিস্তব্ধ রাত আজ
শুধু নেই ঘড়ির টিক্‌টিক্‌ আওয়াজ
আজও খুব লিখতে ইচ্ছে করে,
আজ লিখি আমার স্বর্গীয় মা'র তরে,
রোজ রাতে ঘুম ভেঙ্গে যায়,
নীচে আসি করি স্বরা,
সূর্য ওঠার আগে যোগব্যায়াম আর
প্রাণায়ম করা,
এখন আছে শুধু ভরসা দৈবশক্তি,
দেখো 'মা', মনে থাকে যেন অটল ভক্তি,
রোজ সকালে উঠে সূর্যদেবকে তাই বলি,
'সূর্যদেব' তোমার তো অনেক তেজ,
দাও না আমায় তোমার থেকে কিছুটা
হতে পারি যেন বীর হনুমান
সঙ্গে আছে যার লেজ।
এ জীবনে কোন দোষ করিব না
কাতর হই পরদুঃখে,
মানুষকে যেন প্রেম দিতে পারি
সদা থাকি হাসিমুখে।

To Mother

By Rakhi Guha
(English adaptation of the poem
in the previous page by Sushmita Dutt)

The night is silent again,
Unconquerable.
Sealed silence, monotonous,
Ticking of the clock is stifled.
Time has come to a halt.

It's time again,
holding to arms, urging me
to write. I do feel like
writing, and tonight, it's
for you, my mother,

My lost mother,
I wake-up every night
In an urgency for yoga
before the sun rises.
Yoga, my only strength
I can regain, I think.

And, now, it is you,
mother, your strength
courage and faith
that you instilled in me,
I relay that to the Sun and,
beg for some light.

I bend down on my knees,
and, I swear that I will never
incur any sin, I swear,
I will retain within
wounds and hurts, and
I will dispense just love.
Unconditional love
with an eternal smile.

Mother, please, take me
into your womb again
Give me strength.

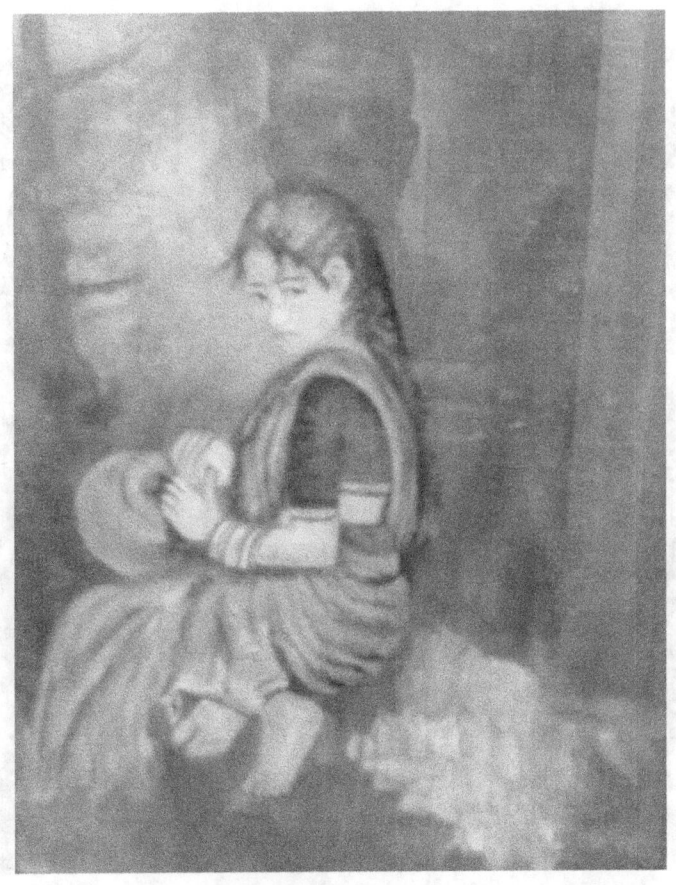

A girl with a water pitcher

Dilip Guha

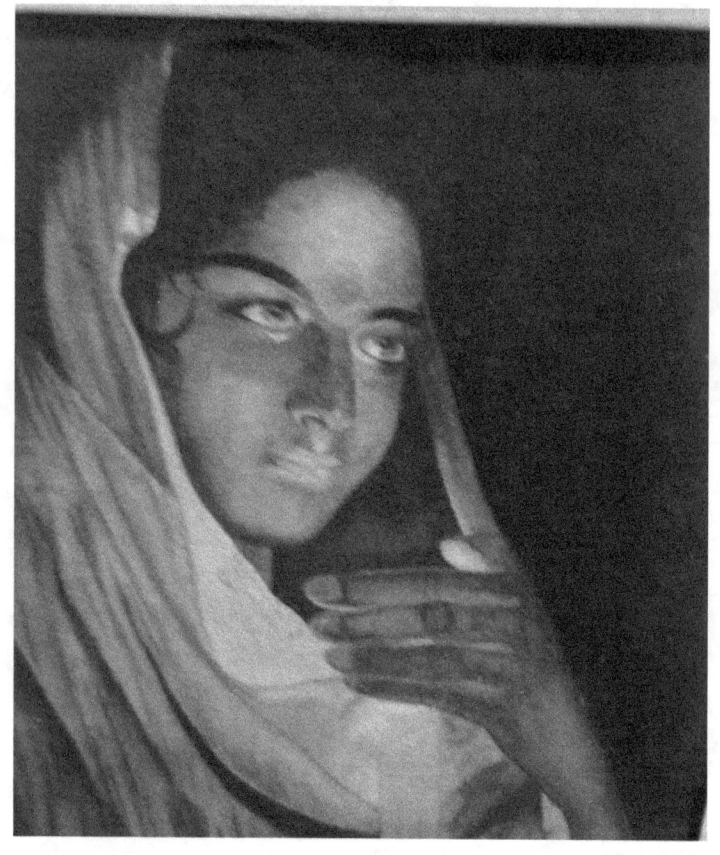

A lady with a lamp

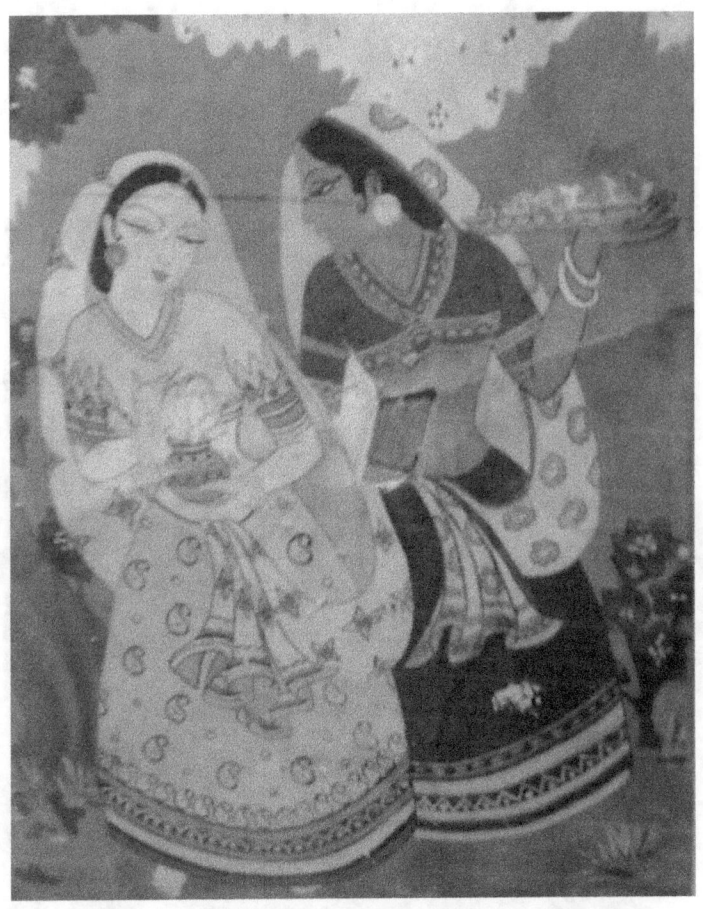

Goddess Radha with another Gopi of Lord Krishna

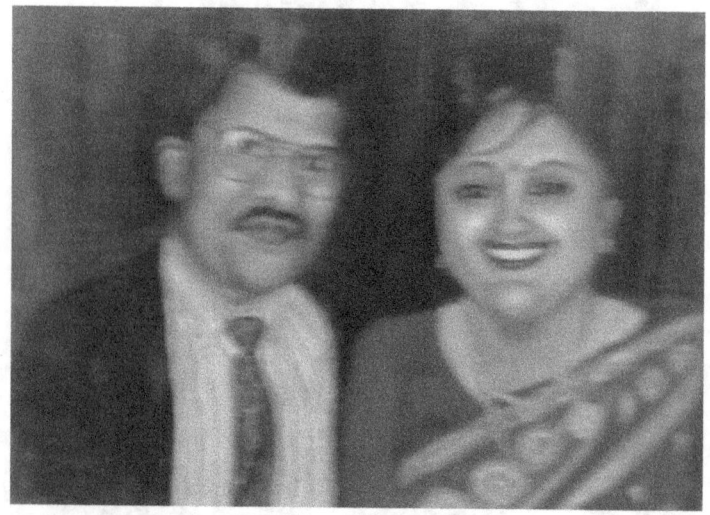

Rakhi and Dilip after marriage

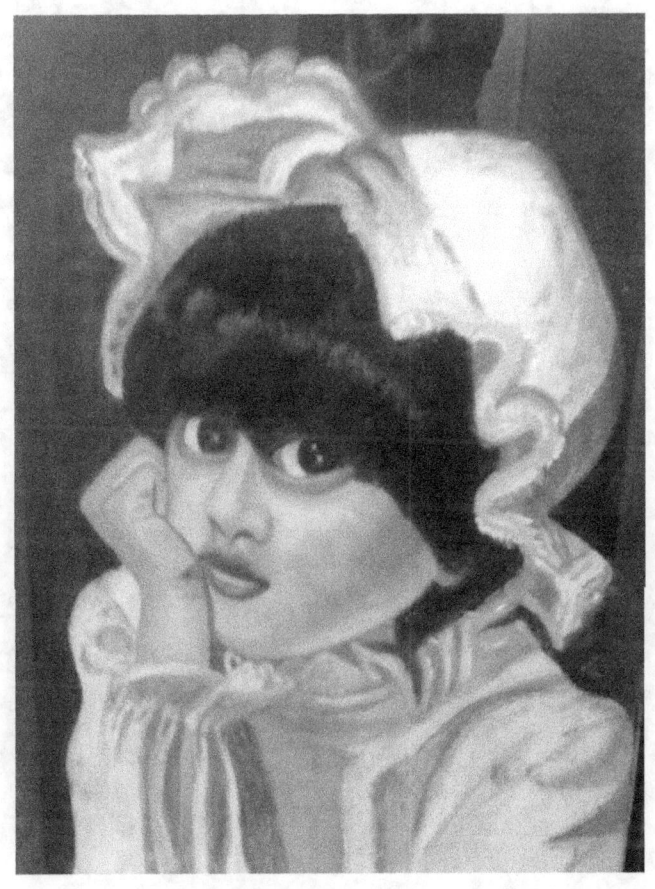

Our daughter, Koel, at her childhood

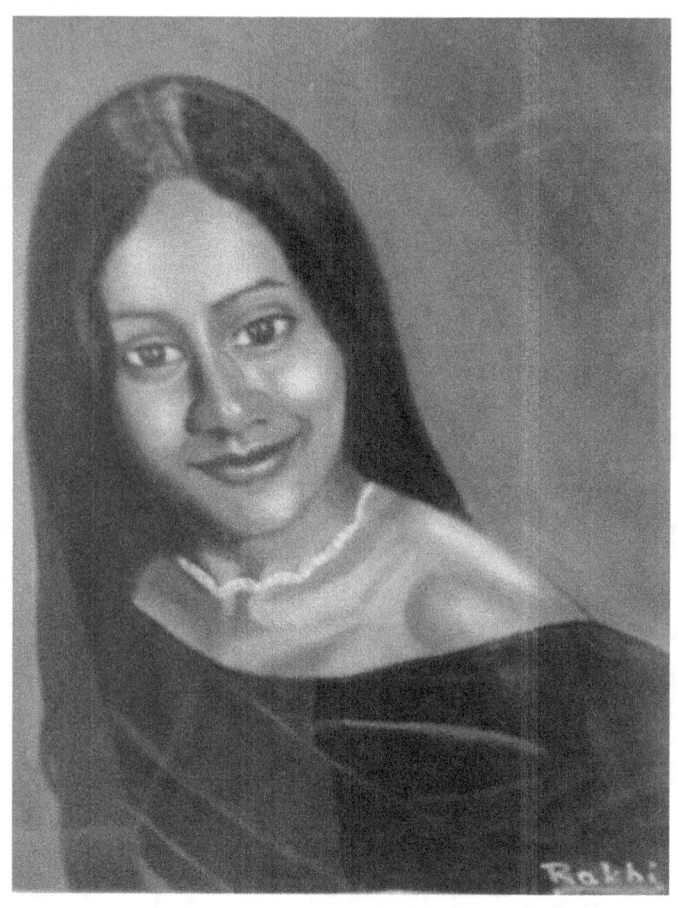

Our daughter, Koel, at her youth

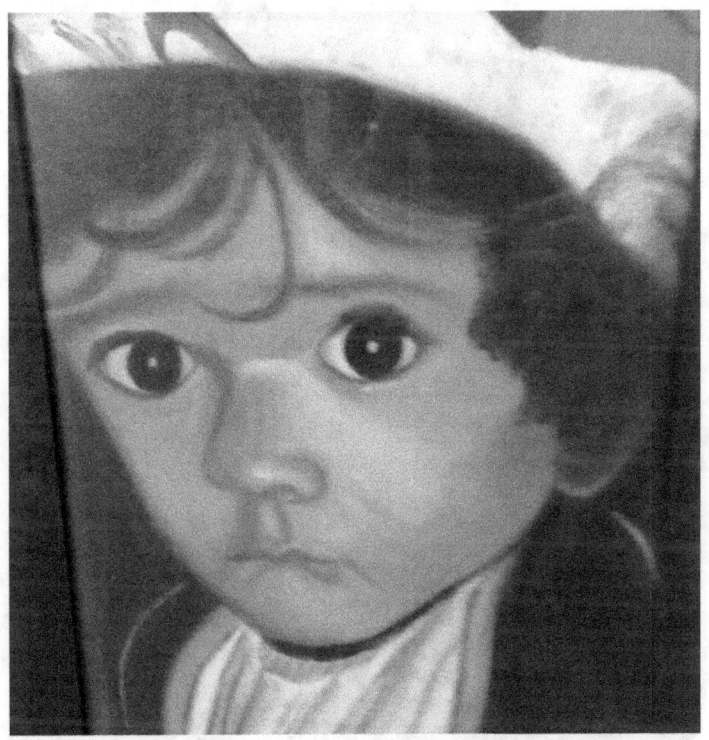

Our son, Roni, at his childhood

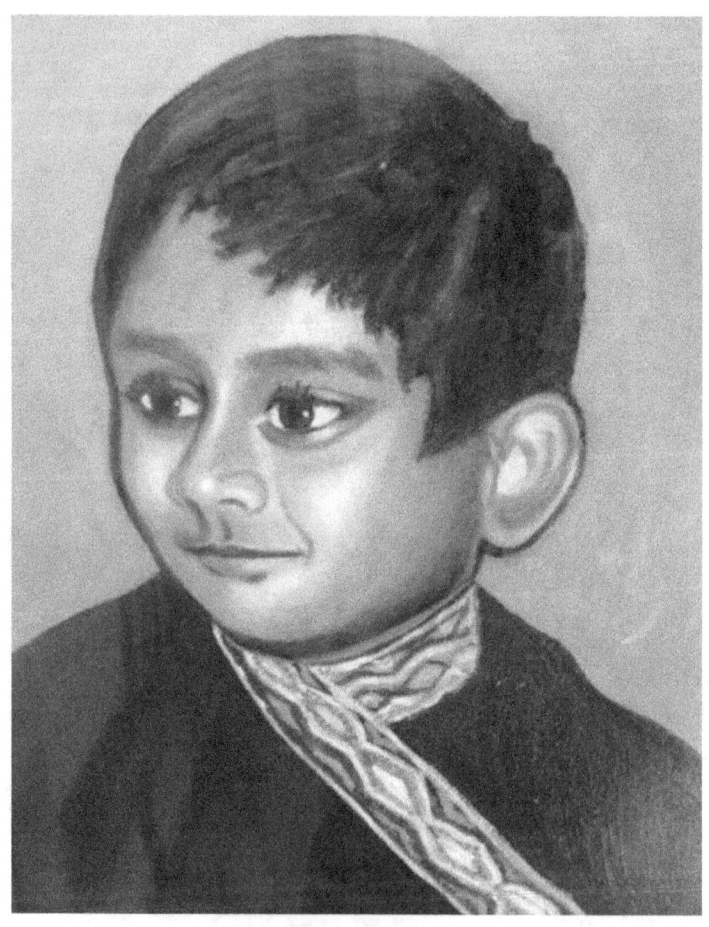

Our son, Roni, at his youth

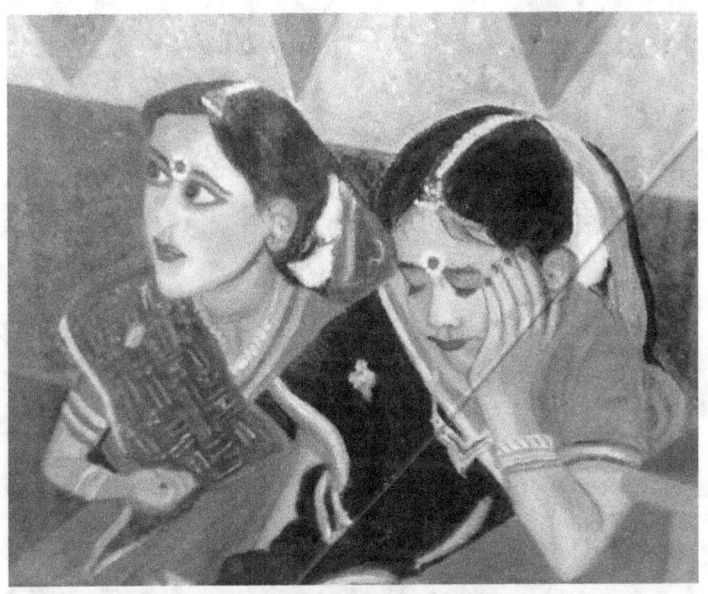

Koel and Sumanta, our daughter and her childhood friend

Dilip Guha

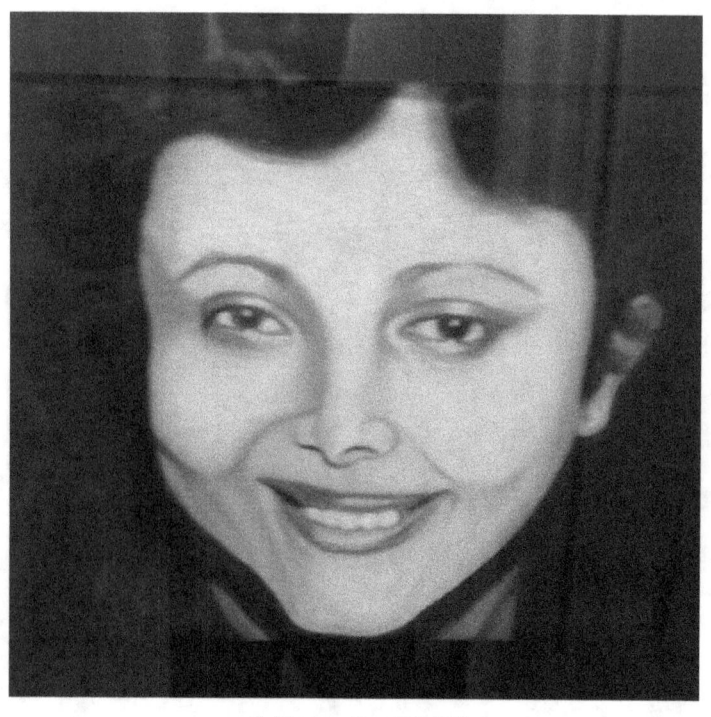

Self potrait of Rakhi

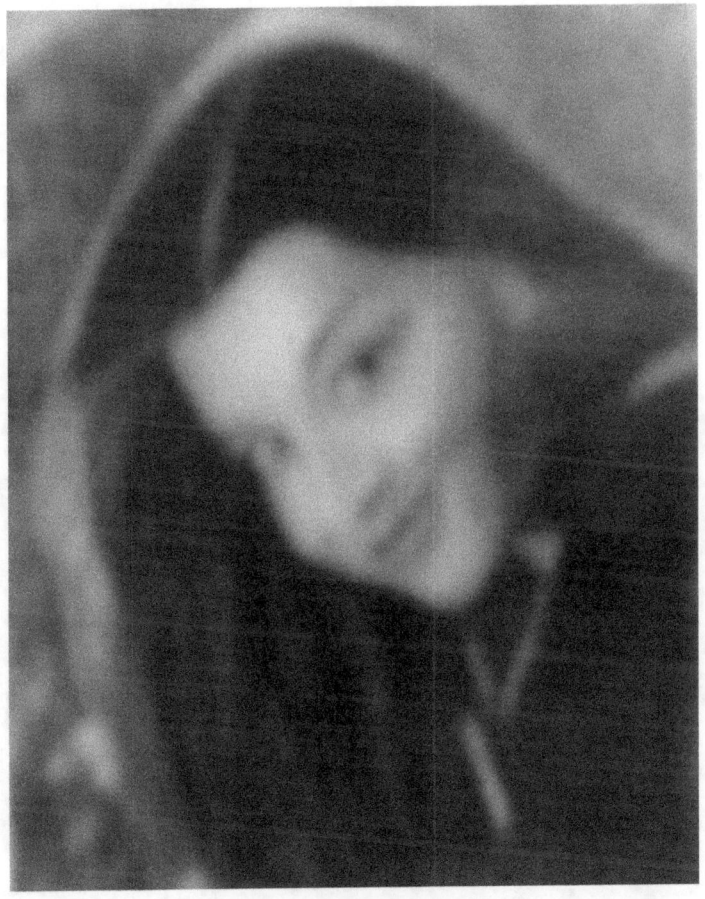

Sohini, Sumanta's sister

Dilip Guha

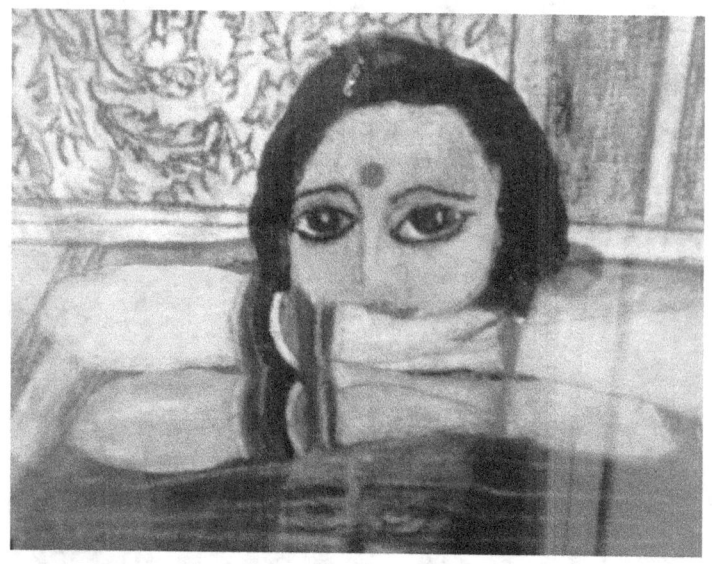

Rakhi's cousin at Kolkata

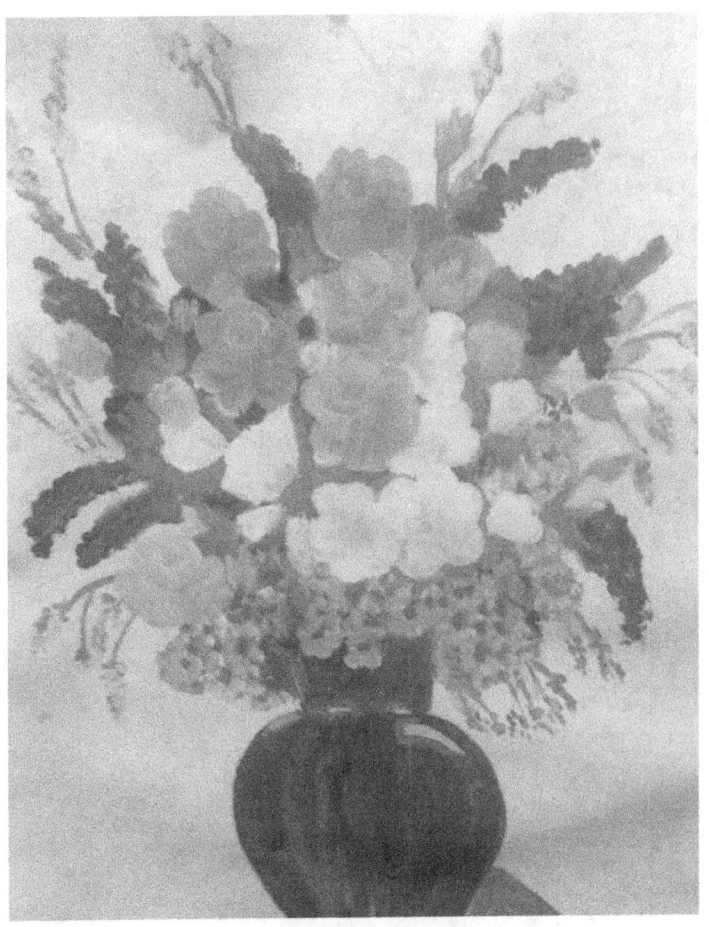

A basket of flowers

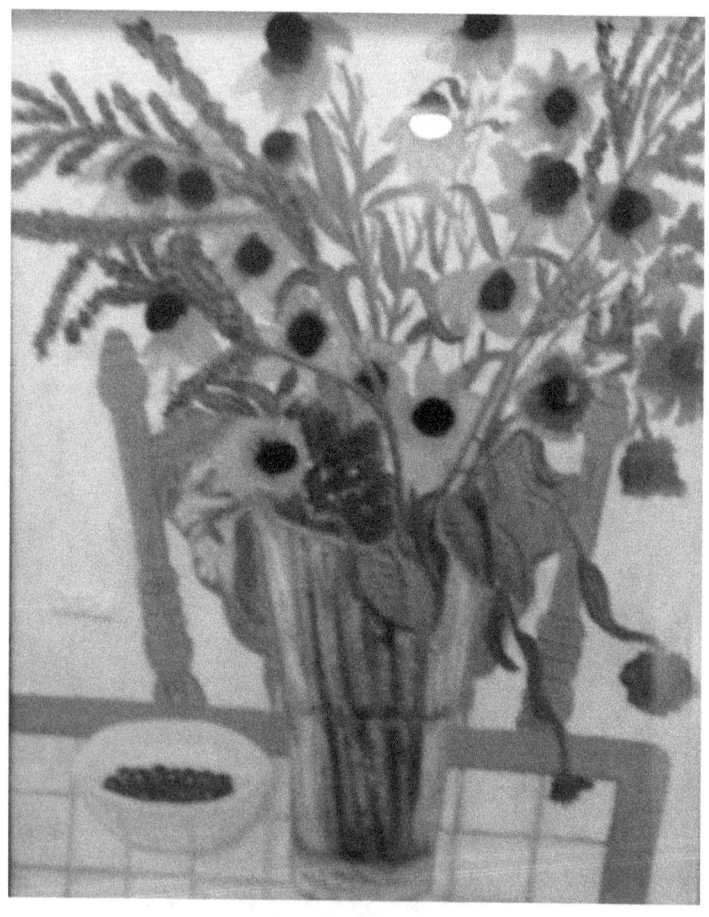

Flowers in the Vase

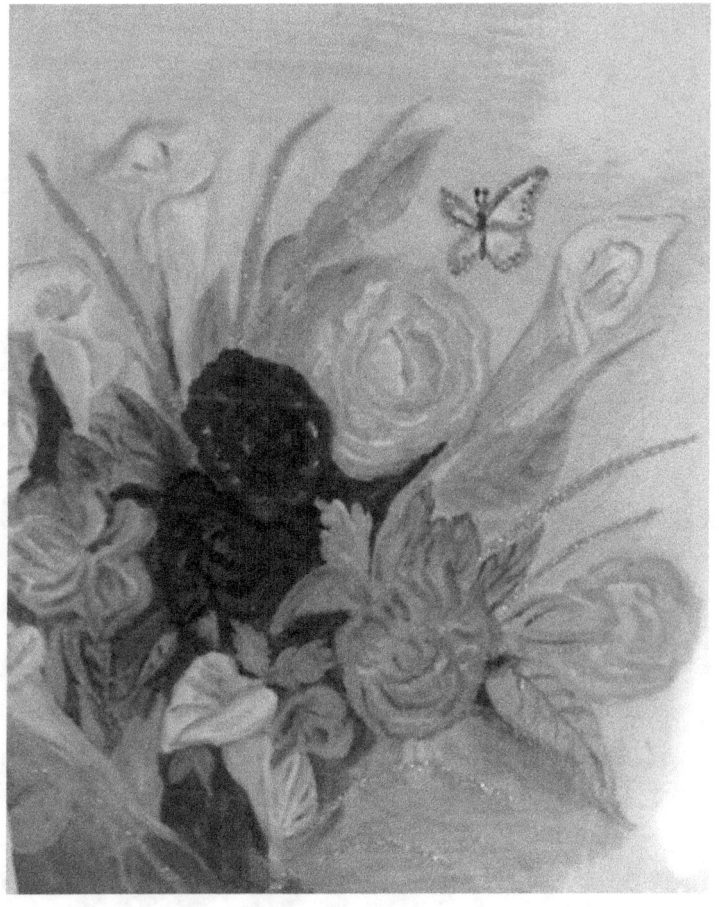

Bouquet of flowers

Dilip Guha

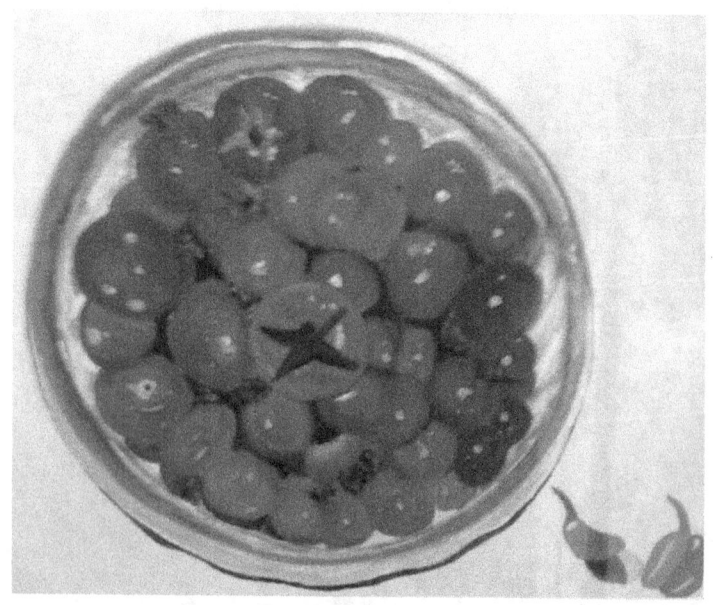

A plate of tomatoes

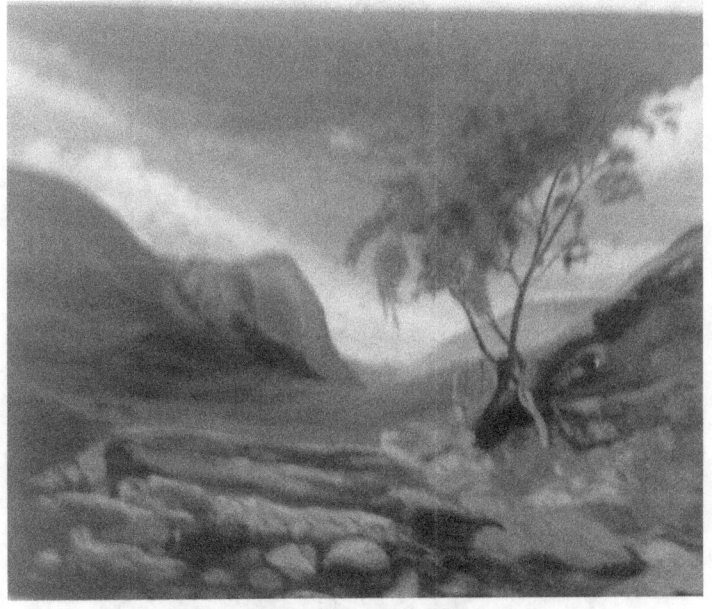

Pebbles in the creek

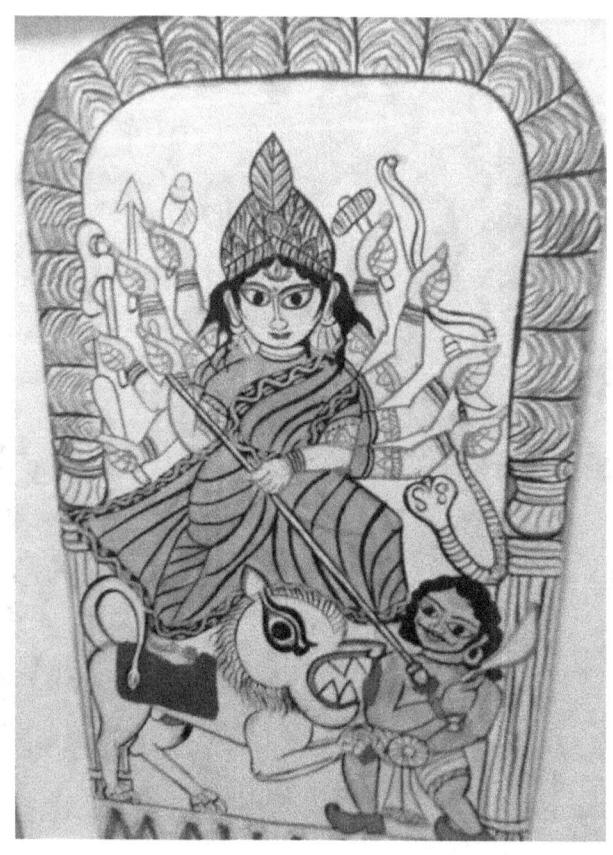

Hindu Goddess Durga - the mother of the universe and believed to be the power behind the work of creation, preservation, and destruction of the world.

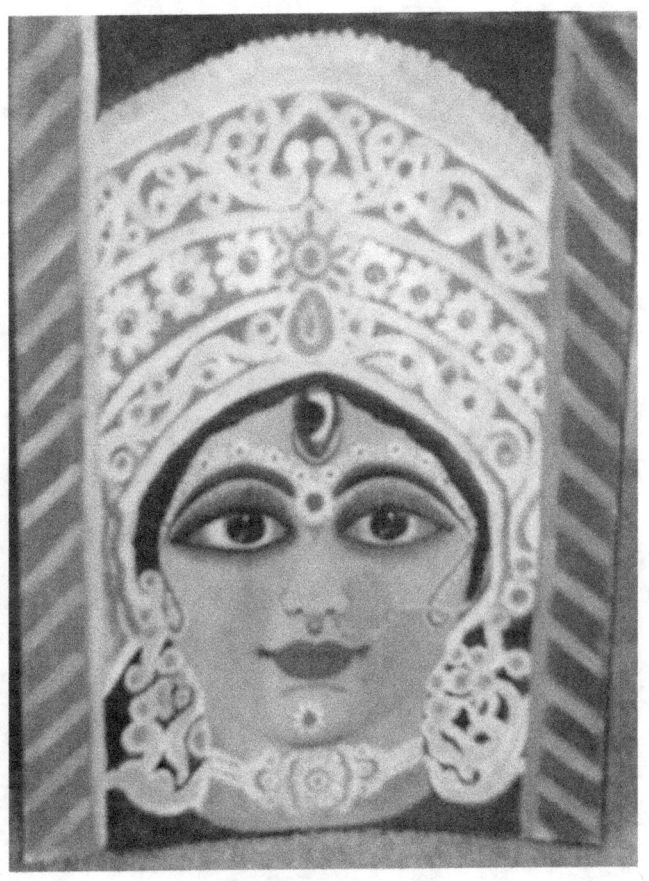

Hindu Goddess Durga

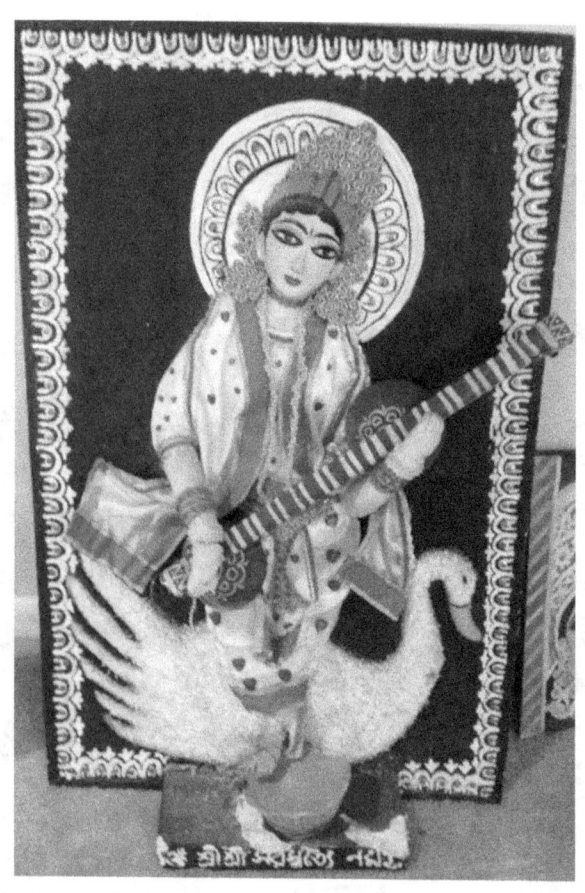

Sculpture for Saraswati – Hindu Goddess of knowledge, music, arts, wisdom and nature.

About the Author

The author migrated to USA in 1975 to get higher education. He attended City College and Columbia University in New York to receive his M.S. and PhD in Electrical Engineering before he joined AT&T Bell Laboratories at Whippany, NJ in 1977. His wife, Rakhi, came to USA in 1981 after they got married. They worked hard to establish themselves and became successful in building private business in their own profession. Dr. Rakhi Guha had an early onset of Parkinson's at the age of 47 and died after long battle of ten (10) years from worse kind of Parkinson's called Parkinson plus or Multiple System Atrophy (MSA). The author has written this biography to share his experience with the patients, the families, and the caregivers who are in the similar situations and can be benefited from this memoir.

The author left his business to take care of his wife full time. Later, he worked as an adjunct professor at Kean University and FDU for a while, and currently works in the public sector as a research scientist. The author has a daughter (Koel) and a son (Roni). Rakhi's legacy lives on through her children. Roni has started college, and Koel is working as a pediatrician in Princeton, New Jersey.